DASH DIET RECIPES

The Perfect Combination to Losing Weight

(Meal Plan to Help You Lose Weight and Improve Your Health)

Mark Miller

Published by Alex Howard

© Mark Miller

All Rights Reserved

Dash Diet Recipes: The Perfect Combination to Losing Weight (Meal Plan to Help You Lose Weight and Improve Your Health)

ISBN 978-1-990169-00-7

All rights reserved. No part of this guide may be reproduced in any form without permission in writing from the publisher except in the case of brief quotations embodied in critical articles or reviews.

Legal & Disclaimer

The information contained in this book is not designed to replace or take the place of any form of medicine or professional medical advice. The information in this book has been provided for educational and entertainment purposes only.

The information contained in this book has been compiled from sources deemed reliable, and it is accurate to the best of the Author's knowledge; however, the Author cannot guarantee its accuracy and validity and cannot be held liable for any errors or omissions. Changes are periodically made to this book. You must consult your doctor or get professional medical advice before using any of the suggested remedies, techniques, or information in this book.

Table of contents

- PART 1 1
- INTRODUCTION 2
- WHAT IS THE DASH DIET 3
- CHAPTER 1 DASH DIET: ALCOHOL AND CAFFEINE 8
- CHAPTER 2: HEALTHY BLOOD PRESSURE IS IMPORTANT 10
- CHAPTER 3: DASH DIET IN LOSING WEIGHT 13
- CHAPTER 4: DASH DIET RECIPES 17
- BREAKFAST RECIPES 21
  - Banana And Peanut Butter Toast 23
  - Honey & Fig Yogurt 23
  - Microwave Egg Omelette 23
  - French Toast 24
  - Veggie Egg Omelete 25
  - Bircher Muesli 25
  - Oatmeal Breakfast With Fruits 26
  - Egg And Avocado Sandwich 27
  - Vegetable Omelet With Tomatoes And Paprika 27
  - Scrambled Egg Spinach And Berries 29
  - Breakfast Avocado Crunch 29
  - Breakfast Oatmeal Delight 30
  - Overnight Peanut Butter Oats 30
  - Express Cereals 31
  - Green Smoothie With Oats Breakfast 32
  - Baked Oatmeal Granola 32
  - Banana Oats Porridge 33
  - Blueberry Pancake 34
  - Quick Quesadilla For Breakfast 35
  - Apple Quesadilla 35
  - Egg Wraps For Breakfast 36

MAIN DISH RECIPES 38

Pan-Fried Salmon With Salad 38
Veggie Variety 39
Vegetable Pasta 40
Vegetable Noodles With Bolognese 41
Harissa Bolognese With Vegetable Noodles 42
Curry Vegetable Noodles With Chicken 43
Pork Chop Malt Beer Sauce With Vegetable Noodles 44
Sweet And Sour Vegetable Noodles 45
Tuna Sandwich 46
Fruited Quinoa Salad 47
Make Yourself Wrap Dough 48
Turkey Wrap 49
Chicken Wrap 50
Veggie Wrap 51
Salmon Wrap 52
Dill Chicken Salad 52
Spelt Pesto Salad 53
Baked Vegetable Salad 54
Shrimp Peach Salad 55
Grilled Tilapia With Salsa 57
Noodle Poultry Sausage Casserole 58
Meat Sausage -Ragout 59
Sausage Potato Meal 60
Grilled Salmon Fillets 61
Rocket Wrap In Honey Mustard Sauce 61
Homemade Bread Rolls With Cream Cheese Salmon Filling 62
Turkey Meatballs With Paprika 64

SNACKS AND DESSERTS RECIPES 66

Brazilian Acai Bowl 67
Easy Acai Bowl 68
Fast Apple Rings 68
Yogurt Berry Parfaits 69
Swiss Rosti 70
Baked Popcorn 70

Protein Custard	71
Wafer Snacks	72
No-Bake Cookies	73
No-Bake Choco Peanut Butter	74
Suggested Dash Diet Snacks	75

DIPS & COCKTAIL SAUCE RECIPES 77

Cocktail Sauce	77
Skinny Ranch Dip	78
Creamy Herb Dip With Raw Vegetables	78
Quick Cocktail Sauce	79
Garlic And Chives Dip	80
Seafood Dip	80
Garlic Dip	82
Avocado Dip	82
Spicy Broccoli Dip	83
Fruit Dip	84
Vegetable Dips For Diabetic	84
Basil Egg Dip With Yogurt	85
Liptauer Spread	86
Raclette Dip	86
Plum Compote	87
Cream Cheese Dip With Bacon	88
Cream Cheese Dip With Garlic	88
Herb Cream Cheese Dip	89

WEIGHT LOSS SMOOTHIES & COCKTAILS RECIPES 90

Strawberry Banana Kale Smoothie	92
Green Smoothie	93
Mango Smoothie Surprise	93
Peanut Butter And Banana Smoothie	94
Chocolate Raspberry Smoothie	94
Apple Smoothie	95
Banana Milk	95
Banana Pineapple Smoothie	96
Green Boost Smoothie	96

Pumpkin Smoothie 97
Chia- Berry Smoothie 97
Spicy Green Smoothies 98
Vanilla Berry Smoothies 98
Spirulina Smoothies.. 99
Belly-Busting Berry Smoothies... 99
Skinny Orange Dream Smoothie 99
Peach Blueberry Banana Spinach 100
Oats And Chia Smoothie 100
Pineapple Pecan Strawberry 101
Lemon, Papaya And Cayenne Pepper Smoothie 101
Mango Yogurt Smoothie 102
Green Mango Smoothie 102
Green Almonds, Apple Smoothie.. 102
Refreshing Smoothie 103
Avocado Yogurt With Wasabi Smoothie 104
Berry Mint Cocktail 104
Pear Ginger Cocktail 105
Carrot & Bell Pepper Booster Smoothie...................................... 105

SOUP RECIPES... 107

Easy Cream Of Mushroom Soup 107
Carrot Soup With Curry 108
Creamy Asparagus Soup 109
Minestrone - Fast And Fresh Variant 110
Barley Soup With Mushrooms 111
Potato Soup With Apples And Brie 112
Pumpkin Soup In Coconut Milk 114
Garlic Veggie Soup 114

CONCLUSION 116

PART 2.. 118

INTRODUCTION 119

CHAPTER 1: WHAT'S DASH DIET?.. 121

CHAPTER 2: WHY WAS THE DASH DIET CREATED?................ 125

CHAPTER 3: DASH DIET EATING PLAN FOR HAPPY HEALTHY LIFE 130

CHAPTER 4: DASH DIET TO CONTROL HYPERTENSION - COULD IT BE POSSIBLE? 135

CHAPTER 5: DASH DIET FOOD GROUPS 145

CHAPTER 6: PORTION CONTROL AND SERVING SIZES 152

DASH DIET FOOD LIST 154

CHAPTER 7: EMPLOYING DASH TO SHED WEIGHT 157

CHAPTER 8: DASH-FRIENDLY RECIPES 166

BLUEBERRY GREEN SMOOTHIE 168
PAPAYA GOODNESS 169
DIABETIC-FRIENDLY GREEN SMOOTHIE 170
BANANA ALMOND SMOOTHIE 170
TROPICAL SMOOTHIE 171
BERRY BANANA GREEN SMOOTHIE 171
PEACH GREEN SMOOTHIE 172
GREEN AVOCADO SMOOTHIE 172
MELON MÉLANGE 173
STRAWBERRY CUCUMBER DE LIGHT 174

CHAPTER 9: DASH BREAK-FAST 176

STINKS USING ALMOND BUTTER AND BANANA 176
ENGLISH MUFFIN USING BERRIES 176
PROTEIN BOWL 177
BERRIES DE LUXE OATMEAL 178
APPLES AND CINNAMON OATMEAL 178
ENERGY OATMEAL 179
ANNA'S HOMEMADE GRANOLA 179
WARM QUINOA USING BERRIES 180
FRUITY YOGURT PARFAIT 181
BANANA ALMOND YOGURT 182
OPEN-FACED BREAKFAST SANDWICH 182
BROCCOLI OMELET 183
CARAMELIZED ONIONS 184

Veggie Scramble	185
CONCLUSION	**187**

Part 1

Introduction

History of Dash Diet

Dash Diet (Dietary Approaches to Stop Hypertension originated during 1990's as Hypertension or High Blood pressure affects a lot of people in US and UK. The National Institute of Health (NIH) started funding for several research projects to see a specific dietary interventions in treating hypertension. Scientists supported by National Heart, Lung, and Blood Institute (NHLBI) and conducted two key studies. Their findings showed that blood pressure were reduces with an eating plan that is low in saturated fat, cholesterol, and total fat and that emphasizes fruits, vegetables, and fat-free or low-fat milk and milk products. This eating plan known as the DASH diet. This includes whole grain products, fish and poultry, and nuts. Reduced in lean red meat, sweets, added sugars, and sugar containing beverages.

The first DASH study involved 459 adults with systolic blood pressures of less than 160 mmHg and diastolic pressures of 80–95 mmHg. About 27 percent of the participants had high blood pressure. About 50 percent were women and 60 percent were African Americans. It compared three eating plans: a plan that includes foods similar to what many Americans regularly eat; a plan that includes foods similar to what many Americans regularly eat plus more fruits and vegetables; and the DASH eating plan. All three plans included about 3,000 milligrams of sodium daily.

None of the plans was vegetarian or used specialty foods.

Results were dramatic. Participants who followed both the plan that included more fruits and vegetables and the DASH eating plan had reduced blood pressure. But the DASH eating plan had the greatest effect, especially for those with high blood pressure. Furthermore, the blood pressure reductions came fast—within 2 weeks of starting the plan.

The second DASH study looked at the effect on blood pressure of a reduced dietary sodium intake as participants followed either the DASH eating plan or an eating plan typical of what many Americans consume. This second study involved 412 participants. Participants were randomly assigned to one of the two eating plans and then followed for a month at each of the three sodium levels. The three sodium levels were a higher intake of about 3,300 milligrams per day (the level consumed by many Americans), an intermediate intake of about 2,300 milligrams per day, and a lower intake of about 1,500 milligrams per day.

Results showed that reducing dietary sodium lowered blood pressure for both eating plans. At each sodium level, blood pressure was lower on the DASH eating plan than on the other eating plan. The greatest blood pressure reductions were for the DASH eating plan at the sodium intake of 1,500 milligrams per day. Those with high blood pressure saw the greatest reductions, but those with prehyper- tension also had large decreases.

Together these studies show the importance of lowering sodium intake—whatever you are eating plan. For a true winning combination, follow the DASH eating plan and lower your intake of salt and sodium.

DASH diet has many similarities to some of the other dietary patterns which are promoted for cardiovascular health. DASH diet is basically a culmination of the ancient and modern world. It has been derived by scientists based on certain ancient dietary principles and has been tailored to target some of the leading killers of the modern society.

What Is The Dash Diet

DASH stands for **Dietary Approaches to Stop Hypertension**. A diet designed and recommended for people who want to reduce and treat hypertension or high blood pressure. It is the lifelong approach to healthy eating. In addition to its effect on blood pressure it contribute to other health benefits. Studies shows that it can help reduce blood levels of homocysteine, a toxic amino acid that may increase the risk of heart disease, stroke, peripheral vascular disease.

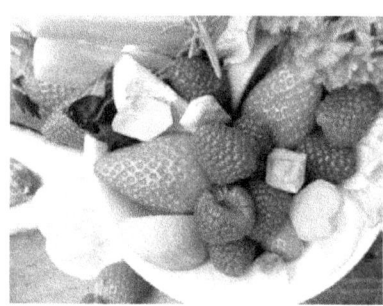

Dash Diet is rich in fruits, vegetables, lean proteins such as chicken and fish, beans, nuts, whole grains, vegetable oils, fat-free and low-fat dairy products. Limiting high in saturated fat, such as fatty meats, red meat, fats, full-fat dairy, sugary foods or beverages, tropical oils such as coconut, palm oils and sodium. By following this, you're naturally lowering the amount of saturated fats and cholesterol. Eating foods that are rich in potassium such as potatoes, dairy (including plain, low-fat yogurt), and bananas, calcium and magnesium can help to reduce the risk of heart disease. It allows a wide variety of foods. You may able to find healthier options for your current meals.

The Standard DASH Diet- program encourages no more than 1 teaspoon (2,300 mg) of sodium per day, which is in line with most national guidelines.

The Regular Dash Diet- lower-salt version recommends no more than 3/4 teaspoon (1,500 mg) of sodium per day

Scientists believe that one of the main reasons people with high blood pressure can benefit from this diet is because it reduces salt intake. Too much salt in your diet can cause your body to retain fluid that increases blood pressure.

Low in saturated and trans fats, Rich in potassium, calcium, magnesium, fiber, and protein and lower in sodium

Based on these recommendations, the following table shows examples of daily and weekly servings that meet DASH eating plan targets for a 2,000-calorie-a-day diet.

Restricting too much salt can be good or bad?

Over the years there are hundreds of studies regarding the salt level for human body that required. Our body cannot survive without some sodium. It is our chief supply of this mineral that is a vital nutrient that we need to maintain proper fluid balance. It is essential for life, regulated in the body by our kidneys. It helps also send nerve impulses and affects muscle function.

It has been known that too much salt will raise the blood pressure. Comprehensive study says if too little salt can also be harmful to your health. According to studies of co-author Andrew Mente, an assistant professor of clinical epidemiology and biostatistics at McMaster University in Ontario said:

"We found that too high levels of sodium are harmful, but also eating a low amount of sodium is harmful". "Having a moderate level of intake is associated with the least amount of harm."

Too much may be harmful, but too little can also have serious consequences.

The lowest risk of health issues and death seems to be somewhere in between.

The American Heart Association (AHA) questions the validity of the studies. It says it will stand by its current recommendation of less than 1.5 grams per day for ideal heart health.

Some trials proven that Dash Diet still better to control blood pressure. Our salt intake doesn't comes all from salt shaker from our kitchen. There are plenty of sources and foods that contains sodium like fast foods, processed, packaged or prepared foods. There are other hidden foods can be sources of sodium like cheeses, salted snacks, pickles, and sauces.

According to Ceu Mateus, senior lecturer in Health Economics at Lancaster University, advises that we should prioritise being aware of hidden salt in our diets rather than trying to avoid it altogether.

"We should be aware that too much salt is really bad, but don't eliminate it completely from your diet."

The most known research is that too much salt definitely increases blood pressure.

You can make gradual changes certain number of servings daily from various food groups. Start by limiting yourself to 2,400 milligrams of sodium per day (about 1 teaspoon). Once your body has adjusted to the diet, cut back to 1,500 milligrams of sodium per day (about 2/3 teaspoon).

These amounts include all sodium eaten, including sodium in food products as well as in what you cook with or add at the table.

The number of servings you require may vary, depending on how many calories you need per day.

Here's a look at the recommended servings from each food group for the 2,000-calorie-a-day DASH diet.

	Servings per day	1 serving is equal to:
Grains	6-8	• 1 slice bread, or • 1 ounce dry cereal,

Vegetables	4-5	or • 1/2 cup cooked rice, pasta, cereal • 1 cup raw leafy vegetables, or • ½ cup cut up raw or cooked vegetables
Fruits	4-5	• 1 medium piece of fruit, or • ¼ cup dried fruit, or • ½ cup fresh, frozen or canned fruit
Fat-free or low-fat milk and milk products	2-3	• 1 cup milk or yogurt, or • 1 ½ ounce cheese
Lean meats, poultry and fish	No more than 6	• 1 ounce cooked meats, or poultry, or fish, or 1 egg
Nuts, seeds and legumes	4-5/week	• 1/3 cup nuts, or • 2 tbsp peanut butter, or • 2 tbsp of seeds, or • ½ cup cooked legumes
Fats and oils	2-3	• 1 tsp soft margarine (non-hydrogenated), or • 1 tsp vegetable oil, or • 1 tbsp mayonnaise, or • 2 tbsp salad dressing

Chapter 1 Dash Diet: Alcohol And Caffeine

Giving up your favourite food and drinks seems very hard enough for people to go on diet, such as alcohol and coffee. Know what's the effect of coffee and alcohol intake on your blood pressure as well as to your overall health. As caffeine and alcohol are allowed on this Dash Diet but you are advice to limit the amount you take not a boundless amount. There are many types of diets that have zero-tolerance policy toward booze. You need also to consider few things when deciding to reduce or cut drinking coffee.

Caffeine

Caffeine is the world's most commonly consumed drink that stimulates the nervous system. Some people worried about caffeinated drinks like coffee may increase blood pressure. Coffee is known that can cause a temporary increase in blood pressure especially those who are not used to it but not in regular coffee drinkers. Some habitual coffee drinkers develop a tolerance to these ingredients as a result seems doesn't have a long term effect on their blood and that don't rise their pressures on one point. If you are worried about the caffeine's effect on your blood pressure, you can limit the amount of coffee you drink only to 200 milligrams a day or about 2 cups of brewed coffee. A single cup of coffee containing 95mg of caffeine acts as stimulant to central nervous system.

For other adults, with normal blood pressure regular cups of coffee (3-4 cups) that equates 400mg or less per day is considered safe. Researchers say coffee drinkers should avoid the sugar, you need to add on skim milk to your coffee instead of using whole milk and sugar. Must stick to healthy and moderate consumption of coffee seems remarkably safe. Those people who already have a high blood pressure need to be more careful and limit with coffee consumption. Ask your doctor whether you should limit or stop drinking coffee. They are often advised to drink de-caffeinated coffee.

Alcohol

Alcohol is allowed on this diet. Although alcohol consumption was associated with reduced sodium it is also associated with unhealthy eating. If you drink too much alcohol it can increase blood pressure and must limit alcohol intake. Heavy drinking can damage your heart. For men to no more than two drinks a day and women to one or less that equals to 14 a week you can't sum it up and have it all at once. Still moderation is the key, as binge drinking can elevate blood pressure that damage liver, brain, and heart.

Chapter 2: Healthy Blood Pressure Is Important

When your heart beats, it pumps blood through your arteries to the rest of your body. The normal blood pressure in adults should be about 120/80 mmHg. It's read as 120 over 80, top number is called systolic while the bottom number is diastolic. Here's the range of blood pressure:

Normal: less than 120 over 80 (120/80)

Elevated: 12-129/less than 80

Stage 1 High blood pressure: 130-139/80-89

Stage 2 High blood pressure: 140m and above/90 and above

Hypertension crisis: higher than 180/higher than 120 (Must see a doctor right away)

Blood pressure is how hard your blood pushes against the walls of your arteries. Knowing your blood pressure is important because the higher your blood pressure the higher your risk of health problems. It causes the heart to work harder to pump nutrient and oxygen-rich blood to the body. If blood pressure is high, it is putting extra strain on your arteries and on your heart. The arteries become thicker and less flexible, or to become weaker. The arteries become scarred and less elastic. These changes happen to everyone as they age, they happen more quickly in people with high blood pressure.

When blood pressure damages arteries, they are not able to deliver enough blood to organs for their proper function that can become damaged. They bring with them a whole range of health problems, such as heart attack, stroke, kidney failure, blurred vision and much more.

As the exact causes of high blood pressure is not known there are several factors that can plays a big role. Like genetics, family history of high blood pressure, age, being overweight, lack of exercise, sleep apnea, Chronic kidney disease, Adrenal and thyroid disorders, stress, too much alcohol consumption and smoking. Lifestyle and diet link between salt and hypertension is compelling. Studies shown that people with high blood pressure are salt sensitive that anything more than minimal is too much for them and increases their blood pressure. Compare with people that add no salt to their diet it has no traces of essential hypertension.

Lower blood pressure thru diet

A well-balanced diet supports a lower sodium that help prevent hypertension and can lower blood pressure in individuals with high blood pressure. Eating rich whole grains, fruits, vegetables and low-fat dairy products and reduce saturated fat and cholesterol. Can lower your blood pressure up to 11 mm Hg. Dash Diet is very important that can change your eating habits.

Reduce Sodium

Sodium is a mineral which is important for the normal functioning of our body. Eating excess sodium raises blood pressure. Scientific studies proven that lowering sodium intake cane be beneficial in blood pressure. The small reduction of sodium in your diet can improve and reduce blood pressure by about 5 to 6 mm Hg. Limiting daily sodium intake is ideal to most adults.

Here's the tips:

Choose foods and beverages that are low-sodium.
Use fresh than package meats.
Choose fresh fruits and vegetables and canned frozen fruits as they are low in sodium.
Choose those labelled fresh frozen when buying frozen vegetables.
Learn to read food labels and check the sodium content on each product.
Reduce eating processed foods as salt is usually added during processing.
Try adding herbs and spices to add flavor on your food instead of salt.
Using low sodium in your diet can control health problems. You just cut back your salt intake slowly and your palate with adjust over time.

Chapter 3: Dash Diet In Losing Weight

Dash Diet is consistently ranked by US News & World Report as top diet and most widely respected diet. It involves making manageable dietary changes that are flexible and rooted in proven nutritional advice. This is the type of diet with virtually no off-limits. This diet is proven to work, some studies found out that people who followed Dash diet had lower blood pressure and LDL (bad) Cholesterol levels than those who consumed other diet. It can also aid in weight loss and weight maintenance.

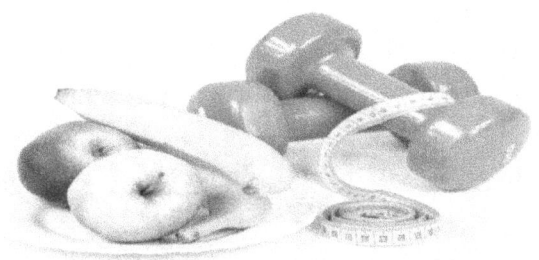

Since Dash diet involves eating fruits, vegetables, whole grains, and low-fat dairy products. It is also some fish, poultry, legumes, nuts and seeds. The main objective of this diet is to limit sodium consumption. It's high in potassium, magnesium, and calcium that counterbalance the effects of sodium that help prevent hypertension or high blood pressure.

Combine Dash diet plan with physical activity it can help you lower your daily calorie and losing weight easily. Moderate-intensity physical activity like brisk walking, running, and swimming or any different activities that you enjoy for at least

30 mins- 1 hour per day is highly recommended. Physical activity work effectively and keep blood pressure at normal levels.

Guides to start Dash Diet and Weight loss

Being overweight or obese increases the risk in developing high blood pressure and many health problems. The Body Mass Index (BMI) is one way to tell whether you are in normal weight, overweight, and obesity. Your weight measures in relation to your height and provides a score in a category:

Normal weight: BMI of 18.5 to 24.9

Overweight: BMI 25 to 29.9

Obesity: BMI of 30 or above

Waist size is also important as having too much fat around your waist may increase the health risk than having fat in order parts of your body. For Female with 35 inches of waist size and Male with a waist of more than 40 inches may have higher chances of disease that related to obesity. Overweight or obesity is linked to high blood pressure in several ways. A large body size can increase blood pressure as heart needs to pump harder to supply blood to all the cells.

Lose Weight Thru Dash Diet

Dash Diet plan was not designed to promote weight loss. Since it helps in lower calories by replacing high calories foods with more fruits and vegetables. It will make easier for you to reach your Dash diet eating plan goals by increasing fruits and Vegetables, increase low-fat and fat free dairy products. Using fat free condiments such as fat free salad dressings, eat smaller portions, choose low-fat dairy or non-fat products, limit foods with lots of added sugar such as candy bars, ice cream, soft drinks, snack on fruits and vegetables or unsalted or unbuttered popcorn or bread sticks and by drinking plenty of water.

In order to get started on Dash Diet and help losing weight fast is to adopt a healthy lifestyle. Most experts agree that when it comes to weight loss a healthy diet is more effective than exercise. Healthy eating that makes the real difference with your waistline. Changing gradually and following guides to start DASH Diet easier.

Here's the tips to get you started on Dash Diet:

Change your eating habits by adding 1-2 vegetables in a day either during lunch or dinner. Don't think of vegetables only as a side dish. Then, try to slowly increase the number of servings to 4-5 to fit in daily.

Limit lean meats to six ounces per day. Focus on increase of servings of whole-meal bread, whole wheat pasta and brown rice. Grains are naturally low in fat. Just cut or trim away skin and fat from poultry and other meat. You just treat meat as one part of whole meal, instead the main focus.

Reduce your intake of calories, cholesterol and saturated fat. For snacks and desserts choose fruit or low-fat foods. Reading label of nutritional facts in choosing foods that are low in saturated and trans-fat. Eating healthy snacks such as frozen yogurt, nuts, popcorn without salt and butter, raw vegetables, low salt crackers.

Add a serving of fruits to your meals or switch to juice or smoothies instead for the whole fruit. Smoothies are full of nutrients and flavor, they can help you lose excess body weight without skipping any meals. Enzymes present in several fruits help dissolve body fat and clear up your circulatory system. Make sure you are adding ingredients that are healthy. Avoid like ice cream, chocolate syrup or powder, pudding mix and sherbet. These have the ingredients that are high in sugar and high in fats.

Unfortunately, as you cannot completely avoid sugar you just go easy on them. Having sugar in natural form is still fine while refined sugar is definitely bad for your overall health. There are plenty of healthy sugar alternatives if you want to reduce or cut sugar from your diet. You may use sugar substitute or artificial sweeteners. Artificial sweeteners such as Stevia (A sweet leaf, Steviva), Sucralose (Splenda).

Artificial sweeteners are known as intense sweeteners as they are many times sweeter than sugar. They are derived from naturally occurring substance- such as herbs or sugar itself. They are better alternatives for sugar as because no added calories to your diet. Great in weight control if you are trying to lose weight. Best for diabetic too as they don't raise blood sugar levels. Still, you need to ask your doctor about using any of sugar substitutes if you have diabetes.

Monitor your salt intake and know how much sodium you need to consume in a day. If you are not sure the sodium level, you can consult your doctor to gather important information. They might have a recommendation for the level that best especially if you. Both version of Dash diet includes lots of whole grains, fruits and vegetables and low-fat dairy products.

Dash diet offers variety of nutrient-rich food choices and number of positive feedbacks about weight loss. It has shown to be dramatically reduce blood pressure, LDL cholesterol, and triglycerides.

Chapter 4: Dash Diet Recipes

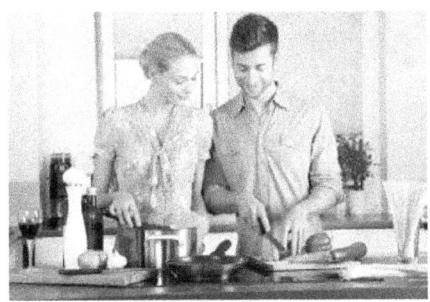

If you want start DASH diet but aren't sure how to incorporate to your daily menus. These recipes will help you get started and as a basis for your own healthy meal planning. Take note that there are some days that just few servings its ok as long is close to the recommendations. More important is to limit your daily intake of sodium as much as possible.

Here's the tips to make it easy for you to start Dash diet:

Choose a Dash diet recipe and you should read thoroughly few times when you decide to make the dish.

Prepare and organize ahead of time by doing a grocery shopping list that you are planning to make in coming days.

List down all the information or ingredients of that recipes. Take note you must stay focus on the essential foods for Dash diet. Spend more time of your grocery shopping in the fresh produce area mostly in the aisles, low-fat dairy and lean meats.

Buy fresh, healthy looking vegetables and fruits. Be selective and don't just simply splurge as it is on sales.

Nutrition facts label of the package of the products that you choose. Remember to always choose reduced sodium and fat. Learn to compare products that has fewer calories. Learn about Label Language:

Sodium:

Sodium free or salt free	Less than 5 mg per serving
Very low sodium	35 mg or less of sodium per serving
Low sodium	140 mg or less of sodium per serving
Reduced or less sodium	At least 25 percent less sodium than the regular version
Light in sodium	50 percent less sodium than the regular version
Unsalted or no salt added	No salt added to the product during processing (this is not a sodium-free food)

FAT:

Fat-free	Less than 0.5g per serving
Low saturated fat	1g or less per serving and 15% or less of calories from saturated fat
Low-fat	3g or less per serving
Reduce Fat	At least 25 percent less fat than the regular version
Light in fat	Half the fat compared to the regular version

Stock up good quality ingredients, fresh fruits and vegetables, low-fat dairy products, whole-meal grains, nuts and seeds and legumes, lean meats, poultry and fish, and condiments, seasonings and spreads. Keep all these food items in your kitchen. Always remember to choose items that are fresh or if it's on canned choose without added sugar. To opt for less sodium and lower fat varieties.

Use proper measuring tools and cookware. Like for example measuring spoons or cups the one we use for eating or drinking is not precise. So, it is worth to invest on measuring spoons/cups and that can be helpful with any recipes. When choosing cookware make sure to use non-stick as it reduces the use of oil or butter. Include also on your kitchen gadgets, the steamer it is important as steaming of will make easier even without oil or butter.

For food flavour enhancement replace salt with herbs and spices. Helpful tips for using herbs and spices instead of salt use the following:

Basil
- Perfect in soups and salads, vegetables, fish, and meats

Cinnamon
- Salads, vegetables, breads, and snacks

Chilli powder
- Soups, salads, vegetables, and fish

Cloves
- Soups, salads, and vegetables

Dill weed and dill seed
- Fish, soups, salads, and vegetables

Ginger

- Soups, salads, vegetables, and meats

Nutmeg
- Vegetables, meats and snacks

Parsley
- Salads, vegetables, fish, and meats

Rosemary
- Salads, vegetables, fish, and meats

Sage
- Soups, salads, vegetables, meats, and chicken

Thyme
- Salads, vegetables, fish, and chicken

If possible research for better alternatives and substitute sodium on each recipe. Try to experiment different techniques you can make spicy food without salt, be flexible and don't be afraid to modify the recipes. Don't just stick to the given ingredients be adventurous, start swapping and use ingredients that you've never tried. You'll be pleasantly surprised at the taste!

References:
1. The NHLBI Health Information Center is a service of the National Heart, Lung, and Blood Institute (NHLBI) of the National Institutes of Health. The NHLBI Health Information Center provides information to health professionals, patients, and the public about the treatment, diagnosis, and prevention of heart, lung, and blood diseases.
2. American Heart Association (AHA)

Breakfast Recipes

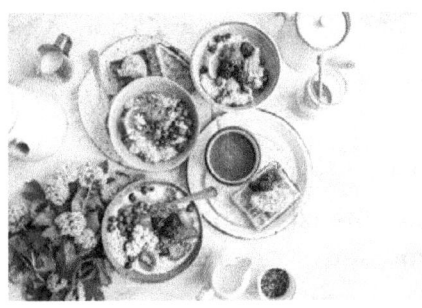

Breakfast is indeed one of the most important meals of the day. Its literally means breaking the fast since you don't consume anything after dinner till you wake up the next morning, your body needs to fuel to start the day and boost metabolism. If you skip breakfast you are more likely to feel hungry and will just grab anything fattening. When you eat breakfast, you are telling your body there are plenty of calories to burn for the day. While when you skip it gives signal to your body that it needs to conserve rather than burn incoming calories.

There are plenty of reasons why you should start your day with breakfast. That includes having better performance thru the day as it increases ability to learn and focus, improves diet quality and are more likely to reach the daily recommended servings for it and benefits weight loss and management as it is easier to maintain weight and decrease risk to becoming overweight. That's the reasons why no matter how busy and pressed your time you must make room for having filling and nutritious breakfast.

If you are trying to lose some weight, eating breakfast every morning has one of the greatest benefits as you can lose weight by just doing do. Studies shows that regular breakfast eaters tend to be leaner. You just have to choose a balanced meal. People that skip breakfast might affect the blood sugar and will lower the tolerance to carbohydrates in which will increase carbo cravings.

If you are suffering from hypertension you should ensure and narrow some basic dietary precautions. Making sure that you are eating healthy breakfast foods that are very essential for managing the condition of hypertension.

Breakfast can motivate you to keep eating healthy throughout the day. Pick a nutritional breakfast to eat and you are good to go.

Banana And Peanut Butter Toast

Ingredients
- 1 slice whole wheat bread, toasted
- 1 tablespoon peanut butter, unsalted
- 1 Banana, sliced
- Dash of cinnamon powder to taste (Optional)

Directions: Serving 1, Preparation/Cooking time: approx. 5mins. Spread peanut butter to toasted bread and top with banana slices. Sprinkle with cinnamon powder to taste. Serve and enjoy!
Nutritional facts: Calories 268, Fat 9.4g, saturated fatty acids 1.6g, Protein 8.6g, Sodium 96mg, Carbohydrate 41.7g, sugar 7.5g

Honey & Fig Yogurt

Ingredients:
- 5 dried figs, chopped
- 2/3 cup non-fat plain Greek yogurt
- 2 teaspoon chia seeds
- 1 ½ teaspoon honey or Stevia (sweetener of choice) to taste

Directions: Serving 1, Preparation/cooking time: approx. 10 mins Combine all the ingredients and mix. Serve and enjoy!
Nutritional facts: Calories 333, Fat 1.5g, saturated fatty acids 0.2g, Protein 11.5g, Sodium 67mg, Carbohydrate 67.5g, sugar 5g

Microwave Egg Omelette

Ingredients:

- 1 whole egg
- 2 egg whites

- 1 low-fat cheddar cheese, cube inch
- 1 tablespoon green bell pepper
- Pinch of pepper
- Ham and Bacon, chopped (optional)
- Cooking spray

<u>Directions:</u> Contains 1 serving. Preparation/cooking time: approx. 15 mins.

Spray microwave-safe big mug or bowl with cooking spray. Combine 1 egg, 2 egg whites and cheddar cheese, bell pepper and pepper in the mug/bowl. Microwave on high for 1 minute and stir the contents. Return to the microwave for 1-2 minutes until eggs are completely cook. Sprinkle with grated cheese on top and crispy bacon if desired.

Nutritional facts: Calories 167, Fat 6.5g, saturated fatty acids 2.2g Protein 18.1g, Sodium 132mg, Carbohydrate 10.1g, Cholesterol 167mg, sugar 1.1g

French Toast

<u>Ingredients</u>

- 2 slices whole meal bread
- 1 egg
- 2 tablespoon non-fat milk
- 1 teaspoon brown sugar
- 20g low -fat butter, unsalted

<u>Directions:</u> serving 1, Cooking time and preparation: approx. 15 mins.

Combine egg, milk, sugar in the bowl and mix. Soak the bread slices in the mixture at least 3-5 minutes on both sides. Heat the pan with butter. Place the soaked bread slices in the hot pan and cook in medium heat until brown. Remove from heat. Serve and Enjoy!

Nutritional facts: Calories 233, Fat 1.9g, saturated fatty acids 1.9g Protein 12.5g, Sodium 67mg, Carbohydrate 32.8g, Cholesterol 166mg, sugar 8.7g

Veggie Egg Omelete

Ingredients
- 3 eggs
- 2 tablespoon olive oil
- 2 tablespoon white onions
- 1 tablespoon spinach, blanched with butter
- 1 tablespoon oregano
- 2 tablespoon olives
- Pinch of salt and pepper to taste

Directions: Servings: 2, Preparation/cooking time: approx 15 mins
Whisk the eggs, add a pinch of salt and pepper. Heat the frying pan with oil and add the egg to cook. Use a fork to gently stir the eggs. Then, add on top onions, spinach, olives and oregano then fold on each side. Serve and enjoy!
Nutritional facts: Calories 175, Fat 14.7g, saturated fatty acids 3.2g Protein 8.8g, Sodium 111mg, Carbohydrate 3.5g, Cholesterol 164mg, sugar 1g

Bircher Muesli

Ingredients
- 100g hearty oatmeal
- 300ml low-fat milk (1.5% fat, possibly 2-3 tbsp extra)
- 1 lemon juice

- 2 teaspoon honey
- 2 small sour apples (150 g)
- 40g hazelnuts

<u>Directions:</u> Servings 2, Preparation/cooking time: approx. 15 mins.

Pour oatmeal in a bowl and stir with milk and let it cover in the fridge covered overnight. Add 2-3 tablespoons of milk if too dry as desired. Halve the lemon and squeeze it out. Put the juice in a bowl and mix with the honey.

Wash apples, dry, quarter, core and cut into pieces. Immediately mix under the lemon juice so they do not turn brown. Chop the hazelnuts roughly with a large knife or in a lightning hacker. Stir apple pieces under the oatmeal. Spread muesli on two bowls, sprinkle with hazelnuts and serve.

Nutritional facts: Calories 175, Fat 11.7g, saturated fatty acids 0.9g Protein 5.5g, Sodium 3mg, Carbohydrate 36.2g, Cholesterol 0mg, sugar 12g

Oatmeal Breakfast With Fruits

<u>Ingredients:</u>

- 3/4 cups water
- 1 cup quick oats
- 1/2 teaspoon cinnamon
- 1/4 teaspoon ground nutmeg
- 1 teaspoon honey
- 4 large strawberries
- 1 small banana

<u>Directions:</u> Serving 1, Preparation/Cooking time: approx. 15 mins.

Slice thinly the strawberries and banana, set aside. In a medium saucepan bring the water to a boil and add the oats, cinnamon and nutmeg, reduce to low and stir occasionally until water is absorbed. Remove from heat and stir in the honey. Place on a bowl and top with sliced of strawberries and bananas. Serve and enjoy!

Nutritional facts: Calories 290, Fat 4g, saturated fatty acids 0.8g, Protein 7.3g, sodium 11mg added sugar 10.1g

Egg And Avocado Sandwich

Ingredients:
- ½ ripe avocado
- 1 teaspoon extra-virgin olive oil
- 1 teaspoon lemon juice
- 2 hard boiled eggs, chopped
- ¼ cup celery (1 stalk), finely chopped
- 1 tablespoon fresh chives, chopped
- Pinch of pepper
- 4 slices whole-wheat bread, toasted
- 2 lettuce leaves

Directions: Servings 2, Preparation/Cooking time: approx. 20 mins.

Scoop the flesh of avocado and place it to a medium bowl, mash' lightly. Add lemon juice and oil, then mix. Add eggs, celery, chives, and pepper and stir to combine. Prepare the toasted bread. Place on each slice of toast with lettuce. Divide the avocado mixture into two parts, spread on toasted bread. Top each with another slice of toast. Serve and enjoy!

Nutritional facts: Calories 183, Fat 4g, saturated fatty acids 2.6g, Protein 6g, Carbohydrate 13.5g, sodium120mg, sugar 2.8g

Vegetable Omelet With Tomatoes And Paprika

Ingredients:

- 1 onion
- 2 small peppers (1 red, 1 yellow, about 125 g)
- 2 tomatoes (about 160 g)
- 1 branch thyme
- 1 clove of garlic
- 1 tbsp olive oil
- 2 eggs
- 2 tbsp sour cream (about 40g)
- nutmeg

- 6 stems smooth parsley

Directions: Contains 1 serving. Preparation/Cooking: approx. 25mins

Peel onion and dice. Cut the peppers in half and cut them into fine strips. Cut stem stems of tomatoes in a wedge shape. Briefly dip tomatoes in boiling water, remove, rinse off cold and peel off the skin. To dice tomatoes. Wash the thyme, shake dry, peel off the leaves and finely chop.

Peel and halve the garlic. Rub a coated pan with the halved garlic clove. Heat the oil in the pan. Sauté the onion cubes and thyme over medium heat. Add the pepper strips and simmer for 2-3 minutes, add the tomato cubes and simmer for another 2-3 minutes.

Whisk eggs and sour cream, season with pepper and grated nutmeg. Pour the egg mixture over the vegetables and let it heat to taste for 5-8 minutes on low heat (depending on how firmly you like the egg). Wash the parsley, shake dry, peel off the leaves and chop. Sprinkle on the vegetable omelet and serve.

Nutritional facts: Calories 200, Fat 14g, saturated fatty acids 4 g, Protein 10g, sugar 6g

Scrambled Egg Spinach And Berries

Ingredients:

- 1 cup baby spinach
- 1 egg, lightly beaten
- Pinch of pepper
- 1 slice of whole grain bread, toasted
- ½ cup berries of choice (blueberries, raspberries, strawberry slices)
- 1 teaspoon extra virgin olive oil

Directions: Serving 1, Preparation/Cooking time: approx. 20 minutes

In a non-stick pan heat oil in medium heat. Add spinach and cook until wilted while stirring often. Transfer spinach into a plate and set aside. Clean the pan. Place again in medium heat then cook the eggs. Stir the eggs to ensure even cooking. Add the spinach and mix, add a pinch of salt and pepper to taste. Serve the spinach scrabbled egg with toast and berries of choice. Enjoy!

Nutritional facts: Calories 221, Fat 10.5g, saturated fatty acids 2.3g, Protein 10.4g, Sodium 96mg, Carbohydrate 23g, Sugar 7.8g

Breakfast Avocado Crunch

Ingredients

- 2 unsalted brown rice cakes
- ½ small avocado
- 1 sliced small tomato
- Pinch of pepper

Directions: Serving 1, Preparations/Cooking time: approx. 15 mins.

In a bowl mash avocado with a fork, spread evenly over the rice cakes. Add tomato and sprinkle with pinch of salt and pepper. Serve and enjoy

Nutritional facts: Calories 291, Fat 20.3g, saturated fatty acids 4.3g, Protein 4.2g, Sodium 15mg, Carbohydrate 26.9g, sugar 3.1g

Breakfast Oatmeal Delight

Ingredients:
- 1 cup uncooked oatmeal
- 1 cup frozen blueberries or (banana, kiwi, or any of your favorite fruit)
- 1 tablespoon chia seeds
- 1 cup non-fat yogurt
- ½ cup non-fat-milk

Directions: Serving 2, Preparations/Cooking time: approx. 25mins

Mix all ingredients in a mixing bowl and mix well. Transfer the oatmeal mixture using spoon into a medium jar, then cover. Place inside the refrigerator and let sit overnight. Serve and enjoy the oatmeal in the next morning.

Nutritional facts: Calories 258, Fat 3.3g, saturated fatty acids .5g, Protein 9.8g, Sodium 66mg, Carbohydrate 47.3g, Cholesterol 3mg, Sugar 19g

Overnight Peanut Butter Oats

Ingredients:

- ½ cup rolled oats
- ½ cup non-fat milk
- ¾ tablespoon Chia Seeds (flaxseed meal)
- 1 tablespoon creamy peanut butter
- 1 packet Stevia or sweetener of choice

Toppings: (optional)
Banana slice, strawberries or raspberries
Directions: Serving 1, Preparation/cooking time: approx. 15 mins

To a medium jar or bowl combine milk, chia seeds, peanut butter and sweetener, then stir to combine. Add oats and stir again. Using spoon press down to ensure that oats have been moistened and immerse with milk. Cover with lid the jar or cling wrap the bowl and refrigerate overnight.

The next day open and garnish with toppings (optional). Serve and enjoy!
Nutritional facts: Calories 299, Fat 9g, saturated fatty acids 1.1g, Protein 13.6g, Sodium 68mg, Carbohydrate 37.3g, Cholesterol 2mg, Sugar 7.4g

Express Cereals

Ingredients

- 1 cup muesli
- 1 medium banana, slice
- 4 tablespoon low fat yogurt
- 1 teaspoon sunflower seeds, unsalted
- 1 teaspoon honey or maple syrup

Directions: Serving: 1, Cooking/Preparation time: 10 minutes

Combine all ingredients in the bowl and mix. Serve and Enjoy!

Nutritional facts:
Calories 421, Fat 5.3g, saturated fatty acids 0.2g Protein 16.1g, Sodium 50mg, Carbohydrate 90.4g, Cholesterol 0mg, sugar 18.2g

Green Smoothie With Oats Breakfast

Ingredients:

- 1 cup baby spinach
- 1 medium banana
- ¼ cup whole oats
- ¾ cup frozen mango
- ½ cup non-fat milk
- ¼ cup non-fat yogurt
- ½ teaspoon vanilla

Directions: Serving 2, Preparation/Cooking time: approx. 25 mins.

Mix oats, milk and yogurt in to the blender and blend in high speed for 15 seconds. Add spinach, banana, and mango until smooth. Serve!

Nutritional facts:
Calories 237, Fat 2.8g, saturated fatty acids 1g, Protein 8.4g, Sodium 22mg, Carbohydrate 46.9g, Cholesterol 4mg, sugar 18g

Baked Oatmeal Granola

Ingredients:

- ½ cup whole wheat flour
- 1 ½ cup rolled oats
- 1/3 cup almonds slices
- ¼ cup honey
- 2 tablespoon unsalted butter, melted

- ½ teaspoon Vanilla extract

Directions: Serving 5, Preparations/Cooking time: approx. 35mins.

Mix honey, butter, and vanilla extract into the small bowl. Into a separate large bowl mix all together flour, oats, and almond slices. Add the honey mixture and oatmeal mixture stirring together until thoroughly combined. Spread the mixture onto a lightly greased baking sheet. Baked for at least 20 minutes at 350°F, stirred often. Serve and Enjoy!

Nutritional facts: Calories 250, Fat 7.8g, saturated fatty acids 3.3g, Protein 5.2g, Sodium 3mg, Carbohydrate 40.8g, Cholesterol 12mg, sugar 8.4g

Banana Oats Porridge

Ingredients:

- ¼ cup oats
- 1 teaspoon chia seeds
- 1 cup non-fat milk
- ½ banana, sliced
- 1 tablespoon dates, chopped
- 2 teaspoon almonds, sliced
- 2 teaspoon cinnamon powder
- 1 teaspoon honey or maple syrup

Directions: Serving 1, Preparations/cooking time: approx. 25 mins

Prepare all ingredients. Soak the oats in water for few minutes then drain, in another bowl soak chia seeds in water for 10 minutes then drain. Heat the milk in the pan on medium heat, add on banana, dates, almonds and cinnamon for 1 minute. Add the oats and cook with milk mixture. Remove from the pan when the oats is cooked thoroughly. Transfer to serving bowl. Stir with honey and garnish with chia seeds. Serve and Enjoy!

Nutritional facts: Calories 295, Fat 3.9g, saturated fatty acids 0.5g, Protein 12.9g, Sodium 34mg, Carbohydrate 47.8g, Cholesterol 5mg, sugar 14g

Blueberry Pancake

Ingredients:

- 1 cup all-purpose flour
- 2 teaspoons baking powder
- ¼ teaspoon baking soda
- 1 tablespoon sugar
- 1 1/3 cups low-fat or non-fat buttermilk
- 1 egg
- 1 tablespoon vegetable oil, (Canola oil, Coconut oil, almond oil etc.)
- ½ cup frozen blueberries
- Cooking spray

Directions: Servings 4, Preparation/Cooking time approx.: 20mins
Combine flour, baking powder, baking soda, and sugar. In separate bowl add buttermilk, egg and oil; add to dry ingredients, stirring until dry ingredients are moistened. Stir in blueberries. Heat the griddle or skillet coated with cooking oil, then pour ¼ cup batter. Turn the pancake when tops are bubbly and edges are cooked.

Nutritional facts: Calories 204, Fat 1.5g, saturated fatty acids 1g, Protein 8.4g, Sodium 87mg, Carbohydrate 35g, Cholesterol 6mg, sugar 8g

Quick Quesadilla For Breakfast

Ingredients

- 2 medium size eggs
- 2 whole meal wraps
- ½ cup low-fat cheese, shredded
- 2 strips bacon (cooked and crumbled)
- 1 stalked green onion, thinly sliced
- Sour cream and salsa (optional)

Directions: Servings 2, Preparation/cooking time: approx. 20 mins.

Whisk the egg in a bowl. Coat the skillet with cooking spray. Pour the egg into a heated cooking skillet over medium heat. Cook until completely set.

Place tortillas wraps on a griddle. Spoon the eggs half on each tortillas. Sprinkle with cheese, bacon and onion. Then fold over and cook for low heat for 1-2 minutes each side or until cheese just melted. Serve with sour cream or Salsa.

Nutritional facts: Calories 226, Fat 12.5g, saturated fatty acids 4.6g, Protein 18.8g, Sodium 346mg, Carbohydrate 9.4g, Cholesterol 31mg, sugar 0.6g

Apple Quesadilla

Ingredients:

- 1 large flour tortilla
- 1 tablespoon low-fat Cream cheese, softened
- 1 teaspoon sugar
- ¼ teaspoon vanilla
- 1/8 teaspoon cinnamon
- ½ apple thinly sliced

Directions: serving 1, Preparation/cooking time: approx. 20 mins

Combine cream cheese, sugar, vanilla and cinnamon and mix until smooth and creamy. Spread on the half side of tortilla and top with apple slices. Fold the tortilla in half.

On a heated skillet or griddle melt a small amount of butter. Place the prepared quesadilla to the skillet and cook until golden brown on side and flip the other side to cook.
Brush the hot quesadilla with butter and sprinkle with cinnamon and sugar. Serve and enjoy!

Nutritional facts: Calories 137, Fat 4.3g, saturated fatty acids 2.3g, Protein 2.3g, Sodium 41mg, Carbohydrate 23.5g, Cholesterol 5mg, sugar 8.5g

Egg Wraps For Breakfast

Ingredients:

- 2 eggs
- 1 tablespoon non-fat milk
- Pinch of pepper
- 2 strips of bacon (cooked)
- ½ avocado sliced
- ½ tomato sliced
- Reduced-fat cheddar cheese, grated

Directions: Servings 2, Preparation/Cooking time: approx. 20 mins.

To make egg wraps: In a small bowl, lightly beat the eggs, milk and pinch of salt and pepper. Pour the half of the egg mixture into the preheated pan. Cover and cook until the top looks set and slightly bubbles about 1-3 minutes. Cook and flip the other side. Repeat with remaining egg. Set aside.

Place bacon on the center of each egg wrap and followed by tomato, avocado slices. Sprinkle with cheese and roll up. Serve and enjoy!

Nutritional facts: Calories 147, Fat 9.6g, saturated fatty acids 4g, Protein 11g, Sodium 72mg, Carbohydrate 3.7g, Cholesterol 19mg, sugar 1.3g

Main Dish Recipes

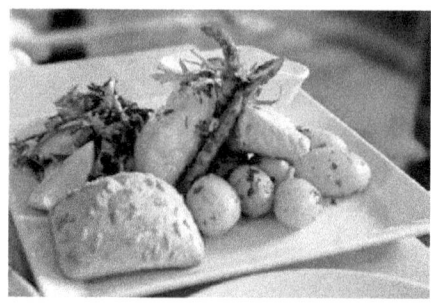

A healthy main dish is an important ingredient to the meal!
The main dish is usually the heaviest, heartiest, and most complex or substantive dish on a menu. The main ingredient is usually meat or fish; in vegetarian meals. If you do choose to add more veggies to a meat dish, double the amount of veggies and reduce the amount of meat.

Pan-Fried Salmon With Salad

Ingredients:

- 4 salmon fillets
- Pinch of salt and pepper
- 1 tablespoon extra-virgin olive oil
- 2 tablespoon unsalted butter
- ½ teaspoon fresh dill
- 1 tablespoon fresh lemon juice
- 100g salad leaves, or bag of mixed leaves

Salad DRESSING:
- 3 tablespoons olive oil

- 2 tablespoons balsamic vinaigrette
- 1/2 teaspoon maple syrup (honey)

<u>Directions:</u> Servings 4, Preparation/Cooking time: approx. 20 minutes

Pat Salmon fillets dry with a paper towel and season with pinch of salt and pepper. In skillet, heat oil over medium high heat and add fillets. Cook each side for 5 to 7 minutes until golden brown. In a small saucepan melt butter, dill and lemon juice. Brush the butter mixture onto the cooked salmon.

Lastly, combine all together the ingredients of salad dressing and drizzle to mixed salad leaves in a large bowl. Toss to coat. Serve with fresh salads on the side. Enjoy!

Nutritional facts: Calories 307, Fat 22g, saturated fatty acids 5.1g, Protein 34.6g, Sodium 80mg, Carbohydrate 1.7g, Cholesterol 20mg, sugar 1.3g

Veggie Variety

<u>INGREDIENTS:</u>

- ½ onion, dice
- 1 teaspoon vegetable oil (corn or sunflower oil)
- 200 g Tofu/ bean curd
- 4 cherry tomatoes, halved
- 30ml vegetable milk (soy or oat milk)
- ½ tsp curry powder
- 0.25 tsp paprika
- Pinch of Salt & Pepper
- 2 slices Vegan protein bread/ Whole grain bread
- Chives for garnish

Directions: Serving 2. Preparations/Cooking time: approx. 25 mins

Dice the onion and fry in a frying pan with the oil. Break the tofu by hand into small pieces and put in the pan. Sauté 7-8 min. Season with curry, paprika, salt and pepper. The cherry tomatoes and milk and cook it all over roast a few minutes. Serve with bread as desired and sprinkle with chopped chives.

Nutritional facts: Calories 216, Fat 8.4g, saturated fatty acids 1.7g, Protein 14.1g, Sodium 140mg, Carbohydrate 24.8g, Cholesterol 0mg, sugar 9.1g

Vegetable Pasta

Ingredients

- 1 kg of thin zucchini
- 20 g of fresh ginger
- 350g smoked tofu
- 1 lime
- 2 cloves of garlic
- 2 tbsp sunflower oil
- 2 tablespoons of sesame seeds
- Pinch of salt and pepper

- 4 tablespoons fried onions

Directions: Serving 4, Preparation/Cooking time: approx. 30 minutes

Wash and clean the zucchini and, using a julienne cutter, cut the pulp around the kernel into long thin strips (noodles). Ginger peel and finely chop. Crumble tofu. Halve lime, squeeze juice. Peel and chop garlic.

Heat 1 tbsp of oil in a large pan and fry the tofu for about 5 minutes. After about 3 minutes, add ginger, garlic and sesame. Season with soy sauce. Remove from the pan and keep warm. Wipe out the pan and heat 2 tablespoons of oil in it. Stir fry zucchini strips for about 4 minutes while turning. Season with salt, pepper and lime juice. Arrange pasta and tofu. Sprinkle with fried onions.

Nutritional facts: Calories 262, Fat 17.7g, saturated fatty acids 2.5g, Protein 15.4g, Sodium 62mg, Carbohydrate 17.1g, Cholesterol 0mg, sugar 6g

Vegetable Noodles With Bolognese

Ingredients

- 1.5 kg of small zucchini (eg green and yellow)
- 600g of carrots
- 1 onion
- 1 tbsp olive oil
- 250g of beef steak
- Pinch of Salt and pepper
- 2 tablespoons tomato paste
- 1 tbsp flour
- 1 teaspoon vegetable broth (instant)
- 40g pecorino or parmesan
- 1 small potty of basil

Directions: Serving 4, Preparations/Cooking: approx. 35 minutes
Clean and peel zucchini and carrots and wash. Using a sharp, long knife cut first into thin slices, then into long, fine strips. Clean or peel the soup greens, wash and cut into very small cubes. Peel onion and chop finely. Heat the Bolognese oil in a large pan. Fry hack in it crumbly. Season with salt and pepper.

Briefly sauté the prepared vegetable and onion cubes. Stir in tomato paste. Dust the flour, sweat briefly. Pour in 400 ml of water and stir in the vegetable stock. Boil everything, simmer for 7-8 minutes.

Meanwhile cook the vegetable strips in plenty of salted water for 3-5 minutes. Drain, collecting some cooking water. Add the vegetable strips to the pan and mix well. If the sauce is not liquid enough, stir in some vegetable cooking water and season everything again. Slicing cheese into fine shavings. Wash the basil, shake dry, peel off the leaves and cut roughly. Arrange vegetable noodles, sprinkle with parmesan and basil

Nutritional facts: Calories 269, Fat 9.7g, saturated fatty acids 3.4g, Protein 25.6g, Sodium 253mg, Carbohydrate 21.7g, Cholesterol 63mg, sugar 10g

Harissa Bolognese With Vegetable Noodles

Ingredients

- 2 onions
- 1 clove of garlic
- 3-4 tbsp oil
- 400g ground beef
- Pinch Salt, pepper, cinnamon
- 1 tsp Harissa (Arabic seasoning paste, tube)
- 1 tablespoon tomato paste
- 2 sweet potatoes
- 2 medium Zucchini
- 3 stems/basil
- 100g of feta

Directions: Serving 4, Preparation/Cooking time: approx. 40 minutes

Peel onions and garlic, finely dice. Heat 1 tbsp of oil in a wide saucepan. Fry hack in it crumbly. Fry onions and garlic for a short time. Season with salt, pepper and ½ teaspoon cinnamon. Stir in harissa and tomato paste. Add tomatoes and 200 ml of water, bring to the boil and simmer for about 15 minutes with occasional stirring. Peel sweet potatoes and zucchini or clean and wash. Cut vegetables into a spaghetti with a spiral cutter.

Heat 2-3 tablespoons of oil in a large pan. Braise sweet potato spaghetti in it for about 3 minutes. Add the zucchini spaghetti and continue to simmer for 3-4 minutes while turning. Season with salt and pepper. Wash the basil, shake dry and peel off the leaves. Garnish vegetable spaghetti and bolognese on plates. Feta crumble over. Sprinkle with basil.

Nutritional facts: Calories 452, Fat 22.3g, saturated fatty acids 7.5g, Protein 37.1g, Sodium 253mg, Carbohydrate 27.6g, Cholesterol 7.5mg, sugar 9.4g

Curry Vegetable Noodles With Chicken

Ingredients

- 600g of zucchini
- 500g chicken fillet
- Pinch of salt and pepper
- 2 tbsp oil
- 150 g of red and yellow cherry tomatoes
- 1 teaspoon curry powder
- 150g fat free cheese
- 200 ml vegetable broth
- 4 stalk (s) of fresh basil

Directions: servings 2, Preparation/cooking time: approx. 25 minutes

Wash the zucchini, clean and cut into long thin strips with a spiral cutter. Wash meat, pat dry and season with salt. Heat 1 tbsp oil in a pan. Roast chicken in it for about 10 minutes until golden brown.

Wash cherry tomatoes and cut in half. Approximately 3 minutes before the end of the cooking time to the chicken in the pan. Heat 1 tbsp oil in another pan. Sweat curry powder into it, then stir in cream cheese and broth. Season the sauce with salt and pepper and simmer for about 4 minutes.

Wash the basil, shake it dry and pluck the leaves from the stems. Cut small leaves of 3 stems. Remove meat from the pan and cut into strips. Add tomatoes, basil and zucchini to the sauce and heat for 2-3 minutes.

Serve vegetable noodles and meat on plates and garnish with basil.

Nutritional facts: Calories 376, Fat 17.2g, saturated fatty acids 3.9g, Protein 44.9g, Sodium 352mg, Carbohydrate 9.5, Cholesterol 53mg, sugar 3.8g

Pork Chop Malt Beer Sauce With Vegetable Noodles

Ingredients

- 1 small bunch of soup greens (about 500 g)
- 1 red onion
- 300g noodles (eg macaroni)
- 4 pork chops, lean meat
- 1 tbsp olive oil
- Pinch of Salt and pepper
- 1 (0.33 l) bottle of malt beer
- 20 g + 1 tbsp butter, unsalted
- 1 Teaspoon sugar
- ½ bunch of parsley

Directions: Servings 2, Preparation/Cooking time: approx. 30 minutes

Wash the greens and clean or peel. Slice celery into thin strips, leek into rings and carrots. Peel onion and cut into slices. Prepare noodles in boiling salted water according to the package instructions. Add vegetables to the noodles 4-5 minutes before the end of cooking and bring to a boil.

Wash meat and pat dry. Heat oil in a large non-stick pan. Fry meat from each side for 2-3 minutes, season with salt and pepper, remove and keep warm. Fry onion in hot frying fat. Deglaze with malt beer, add 20 g of butter and simmer for 2-3 minutes. Season with salt, pepper and a little sugar. Wash the parsley, pat dry, pluck the leaves from the stems and finely chop, except for garnish.

Drain the pasta and vegetables, drain briefly, add 1 tablespoon of butter and chopped parsley to the pan, sauté and season with salt and pepper. Arrange everything and garnish with parsley.

Nutritional facts: Calories 494, Fat 21g, saturated fatty acids 9g, Protein 35.1g, Sodium 520mg, Carbohydrate 38.7, Cholesterol 123mg, sugar 7.6g

Sweet And Sour Vegetable Noodles

Ingredients

- 4 chicken fillets (75 g each)
- 300g of whole-wheat spaghetti
- 750g carrots
- ½ liter clear chicken broth (instant)
- 1 tablespoon sugar
- 1 tbsp of green peppercorns
- 2-3 tbsp balsamic vinegar
- Capuchin flowers
- Pinch of salt

Directions: Servings 4, Preparations/Cooking: approx. 45 minutes

Cook spaghetti in boiling water for about 8 minutes. Then drain. In the meantime, peel and wash carrots. Cut into long strips (best with special grater). Blanch for 2 minutes in boiling salted water, drain. Wash chicken fillets. Add to the boiling chicken soup and cook for about 15 minutes.

Melt sugar until golden brown. Measure 1/4 liter of chicken stock and deglaze the sugar with it. Add peppercorns, cook for 2 minutes. Season with salt and vinegar. Add the fillets, then cut into thin slices. Then turn the pasta and carrots in the sauce and serve garnished with capuchin blossoms. Serve and enjoy

Nutritional facts: Calories 374, Fat 21g, saturated fatty acids 3g, Protein 44g, Sodium 295mg, Carbohydrate 23.1, Cholesterol 58mg, sugar 12.5g

Tuna Sandwich

Ingredients:

- 2 slices Whole grain bread
- 1 6-oz. can low sodium tuna in water, in its own juice
- 2 tsp Yogurt (1.5% fat) or low-fat mayonnaise
- 1 medium tomato, diced
- ½ small sweet onion, finely diced
- Lettuce leaves

Directions: Serving 1, Preparation/Cooking time: approx. 15 minutes

Toast whole grain bread slices. Mix tuna, yogurt or mayonnaise, dice tomato and onion. Cover a toasted bread with lettuce leaves and spread the tuna mixed on the sandwich. Spread tuna mixed on toasted bread with lettuce leaves. Place another disc as cover on top. Enjoy the sandwich.

Nutritional facts: Calories 235, Fat 3g, saturated fatty acids 0.8g, Protein 27.8g, Sodium 350mg, Carbohydrate 25.9, Cholesterol 26mg, sugar 4.4g

Fruited Quinoa Salad

Ingredients:

- 2 cups cooked quinoa
- 1 mango, sliced and peeled
- 1 cup strawberry, quartered
- ½ cup blueberries
- 2 tablespoon pine nuts
- Chopped mint leave for garnish

Lemon vinaigrette ingredients

- ¼ cup olive oil
- ¼ cup apple cider vinegar
- Zest of lemon
- 3 tablespoon lemon juice
- 1 teaspoon sugar

Directions: Servings 2, Cooking and Preparation time: 25 mins

Lemon Vinaigrette: whisk olive oil, apple cider vinegar, lemon zest and juice and sugar to a bowl; set aside.

Combine quinoa, mango strawberries, blueberries and pine nuts in a large bowl. Stir the lemon vinaigrette and garnish with mint. Serve and enjoy!

Nutritional Facts: Calories 425, Cholesterol 0mg, Carbohydrates 76.1g, Proteins 11.3g, FAT 10.9, Sodium 16mg, Sugar 30.4g

Make Yourself Wrap Dough

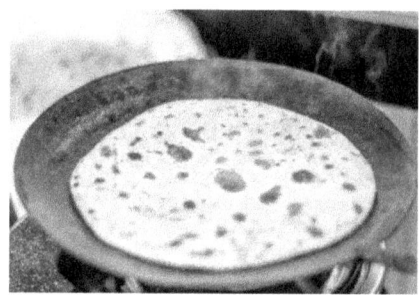

Homemade wrap just tastes better. Here's the recipe for how to make wrap dough yourself.

Ingredients
- 300g whole wheat flour (keep some for dusting)
- 50g unsalted butter
- Pinch of salt
- 185ml non-fat milk
- 1/2 tablespoon corn oil

Directions: Servings 5: Preparation/cooking time: approx. 45 mins
For making the dough yourself, all you need to do is mix butter and milk and heat until butter just melted on stove or microwave. Add the flour and salt to the butter and milk mixture.

Sprinkle work surface with flour then knead for a few minutes until smooth. Add extra flour if the dough is too sticky. Wrap on a cling wrap and rest at room temperature for 30 minutes.

Dust top with flour and cut the dough into 5 pieces, roll into balls, then roll out into about 1/8" or 0.3cm thick rounds.

To cook:

Heat ½ tablespoon olive oil in a non-stick pan over medium heat or lower if you are using heavy based pan. Place on bread on the pan and cooked for around 1-1 ½ minutes each side, pressing down. Enjoy together with your favorite wraps recipes or as naan.

Store the dough in the refrigerator for around 3 days.

Nutritional facts: Calories 237, Fat 3.3g, saturated fatty acids 0.6g, Protein 11.8g, Sodium 68mg, Carbohydrate 56.8g, Cholesterol 2mg, sugar 2.7g

Turkey Wrap

Ingredients:

- 2 slices of low-fat Turkey breast (deli style)
- 4 tablespoon non-fat cream cheese
- ½ cup lettuce leaves
- ½ cup carrots, slice into stick
- 2 Homemade wraps or store-bought whole-wheat tortilla wrap

<u>Directions:</u> Servings 2. Preparation/Cooking time: approx. 15 minutes

Prepare all the ingredients. Spread 2 tablespoons of non-fat cream cheese on each wrap. Arrange lettuce leaves, then add slice of turkey breast, slice of carrots stick on top. Roll and cut into half. Serve and enjoy!

Nutritional Facts: Calories 224, Cholesterol 10mg, Carbohydrates 35g, Protein 10.3g, Fat 3.8g, Sodium 293mg, Sugar 1.6g

Chicken Wrap

Ingredients:

- 1 tablespoon extra- virgin olive oil
- Lemon juice, divided into 3 parts
- 2 cloves garlic, minced
- 1 lb boneless skinless chicken breasts
- ½ cup non- fat plain Greek yogurt
- ½ teaspoon paprika
- Pinch of salt and pepper
- Hot sauce to taste
- Pita bread
- Tomato slice

Directions: Servings 2, Preparation/cooking time: approx. 45mins

Marinade: Whisk together 1 tablespoon olive oil, juice of 2 lemons, garlic and salt and pepper in a bowl. Add chicken breasts to the marinade and place into a large ziploc. Let marinate for 30 mins. to 4 hours.

Yogurt sauce: Mix yogurt, hot sauce and the remaining lemon juice season with paprika and pinch of salt and pepper.

Heat the skillet over medium heat and coat it with oil. Add chicken breast and cook until golden brown and cook about 8 minutes per side. Remove from pan and rest for few minutes then slice.

To a piece of pita bread add lettuce, tomato and chicken slices. Drizzle with the prepared spicy yogurt sauce. Serve and enjoy!

Nutritional Facts: Calorie 348, Cholesterol 133mg, Carbohydrates 8.7g, Proteins 56g, FAT 10.2g, Sodium 198mg, Sugar 7.4g

Veggie Wrap

Ingredients:

- 4 tablespoon dairy-free cream cheese
- 2 Homemade wraps or any flour tortillas
- ½ cup spinach
- 1/2 cup alfalfa sprouts
- ½ cup avocado, slice thinly
- 1 medium tomato, slice thinly
- ½ cup cucumber, slice thinly
- Pinch of salt and pepper

Directions: Servings: Preparation/cooking time: approx. 15 minutes

Spread 2 tablespoons of cream cheese on each tortillas. Layer each veggies according to your liking. Pinch of salt and pepper. Roll and cut into half. Serve and Enjoy!

Nutritional Facts: Calories 249, Cholesterol 25mg, Carbohydrates 12.3g, Protein 5.7g, Fat 21.5g, Sodium 169mg, Sugar 4.5g

Salmon Wrap

Ingredients:

- 2 oz. Smoke Salmon
- 2 teaspoon low-fat cream cheese
- ½ medium size red onion, finely slice
- ½ teaspoon fresh basil or dried basil
- Pinch of pepper
- Arugula leaves
- 1 Homemade wrap or any whole-meal tortilla

Directions: Serving 1, Preparation/cooking time: approx. 20 minutes

Warm wraps or tortilla into a heated pan or oven. Combine cream cheese, basil, pepper, and spread into the tortilla. Top with salmon, arugula and slice onion. Roll up and slice. Serve and Enjoy!

Nutritional Facts: Calories 151, Cholesterol 7mg, Carbohydrates 19.2g, Protein 10.4g, Fat 3.4g, Sodium 316mg, Sugar 3.1g

Dill Chicken Salad

Ingredients:

- 1 tablespoon unsalted butter
- 1 small onion, diced
- 2 cloves garlic, minced
- 500g boneless skinless chicken breasts

Salad:

- 2/3 cup Fat-free yogurt
- ¼ cup mayonnaise light
- 2 large shallots, minced
- ½ cup fresh dill, finely chopped

Directions: Servings 3: Preparation/Cooking time: approx. 25mins

Melt the butter over medium heat in wide pan. Saute onion and garlic in the butter and chicken breasts. Add enough water to cover the chicken breasts by 1 inch. Bring to boil. Cover and reduce the heat to a bare simmer. Cook for 8 to 10 minutes or until the chicken is cooked through. Cool thoroughly. The shred chicken finely using 2 forks. Set aside.

Whisk yogurt and mayonnaise together. Then toss with the chicken. Add shallots and dill. Mix again all together. Serve and Enjoy!

Nutritional Facts: Calories 253, Cholesterol 88mg, Carbohydrates 9g, Protein 33.1g, Fat 9.5g, Sodium 236mg, Sugar 1.7g

Spelt Pesto Salad

Ingredients:

- 250g ready-to cooked spelt
- 100g salad leaves, or bag of mixed leaves
- 100g peas (frozen or fresh)
- 100g Gorgonzola, blue cheese (optional)

Pesto recipe:

- 50g basil leaves (fresh)
- 25g pine nuts
- 40g parmesan cheese, grated
- 1 garlic clove, crushed
- 1 lemon, zest and juice
- 6 tablespoon extra- virgin olive oil

<u>Directions</u>: Servings 2, Preparation/Cooking time: approx: 25mins

For Pesto: Combine all pesto ingredient in a blender and blend all together. Season with pinch of salt and pepper.

In boiling water, cook the peas for 2 minutes, drain and set aside.

Put half the pesto in a mixing bowl and add the spelt, peas and mint leaves, then mix. Stir gently the salad leaves and crumble over the blue cheese (optional). Add more of the pesto if you like. Serve and enjoy!

Nutritional Facts: Calories 446, Cholesterol 7mg, Carbohydrates 49.5g, Proteins 11.4g, Fat 28.9g, Sodium 94mg, Sugar 0.5g

Baked Vegetable Salad

<u>Ingredients:</u>

- 445g sweet potato, skinned and chopped

- 445g brussels sprouts, halved
- 1 bell pepper, chopped
- 1 red onion, sliced
- 1 teaspoon fresh oregano
- Pinch of salt
- Dash of ground pepper
- 3 tablespoons olive oil
- 1 cup spinach or mixed greens, for salad base (40 g)
- 1 tablespoon feta cheese, to garnish

DRESSING
- 3 tablespoons olive oil
- 2 tablespoons balsamic vinaigrette
- 1/2 teaspoon maple syrup (honey)

Directions: Servings 4, Preparation/Cooking time: approx. 45mins

Dressing: In a small bowl, combine olive oil, balsamic vinaigrette, and maple syrup. Stir well until combined.

Preheat oven to 200ºC. Mix all vegetables together except spinach in a large bowl and stir. Add pepper, oregano, olive oil and salt and pepper, then stir. On a baking sheet, spread vegetables and bake for 30 minutes.

Add spinach or mixed leaves in a bowl. Sprinkle roasted vegetables and cheese over the top. Drizzle prepared dressing over salad. Serve and enjoy!

Nutritional Facts: Calories 306, Cholesterol 4mg, Fat 15.2, Saturated fatty acids 2.8g, Protein 7.6g, Sodium 185mg, Carbohydrates 39.8g, Cholesterol 4mg, Sugars 12.9g

Shrimp Peach Salad

Ingredients:

Salad

- 453g shrimps uncooked, peeled and deveined
- 1 cup fresh or frozen corn
- 8 cups mixed greens salad
- 1 cup cherry tomatoes, halved
- 2 medium peach, cut into 1-inch pieces
- 1/2 cup finely chopped red onion
- 4 teaspoons extra virgin olive oil, divided
- 1/2 teaspoon lemon-pepper seasoning
- Pinch of salt

Dressing

- 1/3 cup orange juice, freshly squeeze
- 3 tablespoons cider vinegar
- 1-1/2 teaspoons Dijon mustard
- 1-1/2 teaspoons honey
- 1 tablespoon minced fresh basil leaves

Directions: Servings 4, Preparation/Cooking time: approx. 35 mins

Dressing: Whisk orange juice, vinegar, mustard and honey in a bowl, mix until well combined. Add on fresh basil leaves.
Heat 2 teaspoons of olive oil in a large pan over a medium-high heat. Add corn, cook and stir for 2 minutes or until tender. Remove from pan and set aside. Sprinkle shrimps with lemon pepper and pinch of salt.

In the same pan, heat another 2 teaspoons of olive oil over medium high heat, then add shrimps. Cook and stir for few minutes until the shrimps turn pink, then add corn.

Lastly, combine mixed green salad, tomatoes, onion, and peach in a large bowl. Drizzle with 1/3 cup of dressing and toss to coat. Separate the mixture into four plates. Put on top the shrimp mixture, drizzle again with remaining dressing. Serve and enjoy!

Nutritional Facts: Calories 230, Fat 6.5g, Saturated fatty acids 0.8g, Protein 21.8g, Sodium 318mg, Carbohydrates 24.3g, Cholesterol 165mg, Sugars 13.3g

Grilled Tilapia With Salsa

Ingredients:

- 2 cups fresh pineapple, cubed
- 2 green onions, chopped
- 4 tablespoons green pepper, finely chopped
- 4 tablespoons fresh cilantro minced
- 4 teaspoons plus 2 tablespoons lime juice, divided
- 1/8 teaspoon plus 1/8 teaspoon salt, divided
- Dash cayenne pepper
- 1 tablespoon canola oil
- 8 tilapia fillets (113g each)
- 1/8 teaspoon pepper

Directions: Servings 7, Preparation/Cooking time: approx. 40 mins

Salsa: Combine pineapple, green onions, green pepper, cilantro, 4 teaspoon lime juice, 1/8 teaspoon salt and dash of cayenne in a bowl. Set aside and refrigerate until serving.

Mix oil with the remaining lime juice and drizzle over fillets. Sprinkle with pepper and remaining salt.

Prepare the grilling rack and coat lightly with cooking oil. Grill fillets over medium heat for 2-3 minutes on each side. Serve with salsa. Enjoy!

Nutritional Facts: Calories 167, Fat 4.3g, Saturated fatty acids 0.9g, Protein 26.1g, Sodium 191mg, Carbohydrates 6.9g, Cholesterol 64mg, Sugars 4.9g

Noodle Poultry Sausage Casserole

Ingredients:

- 300g noodles
- 400g pack poultry sausage or meat of your choice, lactose free
- 2 cups soy cream (soy cream cuisine) or other lactose-free cream
- 1 tablespoon Oil or vegetable fat
- Heaped broth (chicken, beef)
- 1 teaspoon curry powder
- 1 teaspoon Paprika powder, pink
- Cheese, grated

Directions: Servings 3, Preparation/Working time: approx. 25 min.

Preheat the oven to 200 °C top / bottom heat (circa 180 ° C convection).

First put on the water for the noodles and cook them according to feeling or packing instructions. Do not cook softly, because the casserole comes in the end for 15 minutes in the oven.

Dice the poultry sausage or the meat and sauté briefly in the pan. Deglaze with cream and then add your spices. I always use herbs of all kinds, curry powder, hot rose paprika. In addition, broth. Stir everything well and let it boil up once.

Put the nibbles into the casserole dish, sprinkle with the sauce, sprinkle with cheese of choice and place in the oven for 15 minutes.

Nutritional Facts: Calories 306, Cholesterol 4mg, Fat 15.2g, Saturated fatty acids 2.8g, Protein 7.6g, Sodium 185mg, Carbohydrates 39.8g, Cholesterol 4mg, Sugars 6.4g

Meat Sausage -Ragout

Ingredients

- 600g Potato
- 400g Pork sausage (poultry)
- 300ml chicken stock
- 400ml non-fat milk
- 30g butter
- 30g whole meal, Flour
- 1 Onion
- 1 Garlic cloves
- 2 Teaspoons Mustard (Dijon or Dijon Garlic Parsley)
- 2 tbsp mixed herbs
- Pinch of salt
- Dash Pepper
- Dash Nutmeg
- Dash cayenne pepper
- Chilli flakes

Directions: Servings 7, Preparation/cooking time: approx. 45 min.

Cook the potatoes as jacket potatoes. Meanwhile, cut the meat sausage into cubes. Peel off onion and garlic, dice small. Put the butter with onion and garlic cubes in a large pot omit - the onion should not take any color, but really only briefly in the melted butter a little glassy. Dust the flour and sweat briefly. Stir in the chicken stock and milk with the whisk and bring to a boil while stirring constantly. Turn down the heat and simmer briefly. Stir in the meat sausage cubes, then add mustard, herbs and spices and season to taste.

Now peel and dice the potatoes and add to the ragout. Just let it stir in, but do not cook anymore. Serve hot.

Tip: add some milk or broth if the sauce is too thick. Enjoy!

Nutritional facts: Calories 358, Fat 20.6g, saturated fatty acids 7.1g, Protein 16.7g, Sodium 555mg, Carbohydrate 24.7g, Cholesterol 55mg, sugar 13.8g

Sausage Potato Meal

Ingredients

- 750g Potato
- 250g poultry sausage
- 1 bunchGreens (celery, carrots, leeks, parsley)
- 1 Onion
- 1 tablespoon vegetable oil
- 30g unsalted butter
- 2 bay leaves
- Pinch of salt and pepper

Directions: Servings 5, Preparation/Cooking time: approx. 30 min.

Peel the potatoes and cut into cubes, dice the celery, slightly smaller than the potato cubes. Peel the onion and chop finely.

Heat some oil in a large saucepan and then add the butter. When the butter has melted, sauté the potatoes, celery and onions in the pot for about 5 minutes.

Meanwhile, peel the carrots and cut them into small pieces, roughly the size of the potatoes. Also cut the leek small. Put everything in the pot and sauté for another 5 minutes. Now fill the pot with water until the vegetables are well covered. Add the bay leaves and season with salt and pepper. Let the soup simmer for about 20 minutes.

Meanwhile, roll the poultry sausage and chop the parsley. Add both at the end of the soup.

Nutritional facts: Calories 271, Fat 13.4g, saturated fatty acids 5.1g, Protein 11.5g, Sodium 392mg, Carbohydrate 27.2g, Cholesterol 51mg, sugar 8g

Grilled Salmon Fillets

Ingredients:
- 4 Salmon fillets (170g each)
- 1 lemon, cut into wedges
- Pinch of pepper
- 1 bunch fresh dill (1/4 cup), minced
- 4 cloves garlic, peeled and minced

Directions: Servings 4, Preparation/Cooking time: approx. 35 mins.

Preheat oven to 400 °F top grill. Prepare the baking dish and coat with non-stick cooking spray. Place the salmon fillets in the baking dish. Squeeze ½ lemon juice over each fillet. Then, sprinkle with black pepper, dill, and garlic. Put inside the oven and bake until salmon is opaque in the center for about 20-25 minutes. Serve with the remaining lemon wedges on the sides. Enjoy!

Nutritional facts: Calories 255, Fat 11.3g, saturated fatty acids 1.6g, Protein 35.8g, Sodium 95mg, Carbohydrate 4.1g, Cholesterol 78mg, Sugar 0.4g

Rocket Wrap In Honey Mustard Sauce

Ingredients

- 2 tbsp mustard
- 2 Teaspoons Ketchup
- 1 teaspoon balsamic
- 1 tbsp honey
- 2 Teaspoons extra virgin olive oil
- 4 whole meal wraps
- 300g poultry sausage
- 1 pinch pepper
- 4 stripes Pepper (s), red

<u>Directions:</u> Servings 4, Preparation/cooking time: approx. 25 min.

Mix mustard, ketchup, balsamic vinegar, honey and 1 teaspoon of olive oil in a bowl until all ingredients are evenly distributed. Especially the honey takes a little more time to dissolve.

Heat the wraps in a pan or in the oven. Place the chicken sliced in the middle of the hot wraps and season with pepper.

Drizzle with a little olive oil and sprinkle with oregano. Add the honey mustard sauce and distribute evenly.

Now garnish with rocket and paprika and roll up. To fix the wraps, use a toothpick if necessary.

Cut the rocket wraps in the middle and serve – Serve and Enjoy!

Nutritional facts: Contains 4 servings. Calories 329, Fat 15.4g, saturated fatty acids 3.7g, Protein 25.5g, Sodium 392mg, Carbohydrate 24.7g, Cholesterol 55mg, sugar 6g

Homemade Bread Rolls With Cream Cheese Salmon Filling

<u>Ingredients</u>

- 25 g of fresh yeast
- 20g of sugar

- 50g butter
- 250 ml of milk
- Peel of 1/2 organic lemon
- ½ cucumber
- 600g of flour
- 2 Medium size eggs
- 1 tbsp sesame seeds
- 150g smoked salmon
- 200g double cream cream cheese
- 1 bunch dill
- Pinch of Pepper
- Pinch of Salt

Directions: Servings 4, Preparation/cooking time: approx. 45-60 minutes

Stir the yeast and sugar until liquid. Heat butter and milk. Add 125 ml of water and allow to cool lukewarm. Put salt, flour and 1 egg in a bowl. Add milk mixture. Add yeast mixture and knead immediately in 6-8 minutes to an elastic dough. Cover in a warm place for about 45 minutes.

Knead dough again. Divide into 9 equal pieces and shape into balls. Arrange on a greased baking tray in three rows so that the balls are just touching. Cover and let rise for about 20 minutes until the volume has doubled.

Whisk 1 egg and brush rolls with it. Sprinkle with sesame. Bake for 15-20 minutes in the preheated oven (electric cooker: 200 ° C / circulating air: 175 ° C / gas: see manufacturer) and allow to cool.

Cut smoked salmon into small pieces. Mix with cream cheese, dill and lemon peel. Season with pepper. Cut the bread horizontally and coat the lower half with 2/3 of the cream cheese. Slice the cucumber and place it on top. Spread the rest of the cream cheese on the cut side of the other half of the bread and put the bread together.

Nutritional facts: Calories 487, Fat 14.9g, saturated fatty acids 3.7g, Protein 18.8g, Sodium 392mg, Carbohydrate 24.7g, Cholesterol 43mg, sugar 3.1g

Turkey Meatballs With Paprika

Ingredients

- 1 red pepper (about 200 g)
- 1 onion (about 40 g)
- 1 clove of garlic
- 6 stems parsley
- 400g ground turkey
- 2 tsp bread crumbs
- 3 tbsp low fat quark
- Pinch salt
- Pinch pepper
- Dash cayenne pepper
- 1 tbsp rapeseed oil

Directions: servings 4, Preparation/cooking time: approx. 25mins.

Wash and quarter the core of the pepper, dice very finely. Peel onion and garlic and chop finely. Prepare garlic properly.

Wash parsley, shake dry, peel off leaves and finely chop with a large knife.

Mix the peppers, onions, garlic and parsley with minced meat, bread crumbs and cottage cheese in a bowl thoroughly. Season with salt, pepper and cayenne pepper.

Form the minced meat into 24 small balls. Heat the oil in a large non-stick pan. Fry the balls crispy over medium heat in about 10 minutes, drain on kitchen paper and serve warm or cold. Serve and enjoy!

Nutritional facts: Calories 283, Fat 15.5g, saturated fatty acids 2.1g, Protein 32.2g, Sodium 165mg, Carbohydrate 8g, Cholesterol 43mg, sugar 3.4g

Snacks And Desserts Recipes

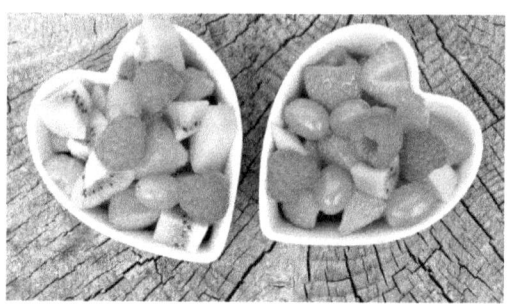

The Good news is you can eat desserts while using the dash diet. This sweet treat is healthy and actually tastes good. Rather than skipping desserts, eating small portions or deciding not to touch the carbs. These DASH diet snacks and desserts that you can eat it in two healthy snacks—one midmorning and another between lunch and dinner.

Brazilian Acai Bowl

Ingredients:

- 2 teaspoon acai powder or 1 packet of Acai puree (broken into small pieces)
- 5 pieces ice cubes
- 1 cup frozen mixed berries
- 1 ripe banana, frozen
- 4 tablespoon rolled oats
- 2/3 cup rice milk
- 1 teaspoon honey/maple syrup or Stevia (sweetener of choice)

Suggested Toppings:

- Chia seeds
- Fruits (mango), sliced
- Nuts like slice almonds

Directions: Servings: 2 Preparations/Cooking time: approx. 20 mins

Freeze ripe Banana in advance for at least 2 hours. If using Acai powder blend to 5 pieces of ice cubes in a heavy-duty blender. Then add all the remaining ingredients together with the frozen banana and blend well to ice cream consistency or until smooth. Serve in a bowl and garnish with your favorite toppings. Enjoy!

Nutritional facts: Calories 201, Fat 3.3g, saturated fatty acids 1.2g, Protein 2.6g, Sodium 35mg, Carbohydrate 41.1g, Cholesterol 0mg, sugars 12.3g

Easy Acai Bowl

Ingredients:

1 frozen packet of acai puree
1 cup plain non-fat Greek yogurt
½ cup frozen blueberries

Toppings:

Blackberries, strawberries, raspberries
Almonds unsalted, chopped

Directions: Servings 2, Preparation/Cooking time: approx. 15 minutes

Break frozen acai puree into small pieces. Blend together with frozen blueberries until smooth. Transfer to a bowl and garnish with toppings. Serve and Enjoy!

Nutritional facts: Calories 106, Fat 1.6g, saturated fatty acids 0.3g, Protein 6.3g, Sodium 52mg, Carbohydrate 21.4g, Cholesterol 3mg, sugars 5.6g

Fast Apple Rings

Ingredients:

2 Apples (big, friable)
1 teaspoon lemon juice
Cooking oil for Frying (choices of Canola oil, Corn oil, Soybean oil and Olive oil)

Ingredients for the dough
- 250g Flour

- Pinch of salt
- 200ml non-fat milk
- 2 medium eggs

Directions: servings 2, Preparation/cooking time: approx. 20 mins.
Place the flour in a bowl, add salt, milk and egg to it, stir well so that a thick dough is formed.
Cut the apples into rings about 1 cm thick, peel them and remove the core. Drizzle lightly with lemon.
In a pan, let the oil get hot. Dip the apple rings in the dough and fry in the hot oil. Turn it over once, as soon as it is nice and golden, remove it from the pan and drain it on kitchen paper. Dust with icing sugar (optional) while still hot. Serve and Enjoy!
Nutritional facts: Contains 4 servings. Calories 240, Fat 6.5g, saturated fatty acids 1.3, Protein 8.9g, Sodium 100mg, Carbohydrate 39.9g, Cholesterol 83mg, sugars 19.4g

Yogurt Berry Parfaits

Ingredients:
- 32-ounce non-fat yogurt
- 16- ounce mixed frozen berries
- 1-2 cups of Granola
- Honey to taste (optional)

Directions: Servings 4, Preparation/Cooking: approx. 15 mins
In a medium mason jar, layer yogurt, berries, then lastly add granola. Refrigerate overnight. Perfect for snacks or breakfast. Serve and Enjoy!
Nutritional information: Calories 298, Fat 1.7g, saturated fatty acids 0.3g, Protein 16.1g, Sodium 129mg, Carbohydrate 53.6g, Cholesterol 7mg, Sugars 18g

Swiss Rosti

Ingredients
- 500g Potatoes (floury)
- 1 small onion
- Pinch of salt and pepper
- 3 tablespoons unsalted low-fat butter

Directions: servings 4, Preparation/cooking time: approx. 25 mins.
Peel and finely grate the potatoes, peel the onion and finely chop. Mix the potatoes with the onions, salt and pepper.
Heat the butter in a pan, add a tablespoon of small rösti to the pan and press flat, sauté the rösti well, then turn over and fry until crispy from the other side. Drain the rösti on the kitchen paper and serve hot.
Nutritional information: Contains 4 servings. Calories 248, Fat 6.4g, saturated fatty acids 3.9, Protein 4.9g, Sodium 96mg, Carbohydrate 44.5g, Cholesterol 16mg, Sugars 3.3g
Tips on the recipe
The Rösti are ideal as a snack in between or as a main meal with a fresh sour cream dip

Baked Popcorn

Ingredients:

- 8 cups of popcorn unsalted
- 3 tablespoon maple syrup
- 2 tablespoon of coconut oil
- 3 tablespoons of brown sugar
- 3 tablespoon of Hemp seeds
- 3 tablespoon of Chai seeds
- ¼ teaspoon of ground nutmeg

- Pinch of salt

Directions: Servings 5, Preparation/Cooking time: approx. 35 mins
Line baking sheet with parchment paper. Preheat oven to 275 degrees. In a large bowl place popcorn. Dizzle with maple syrup and coconut oil then toss to coat.
Mix sugar, 1 ½ tablespoon hemp seeds, 1 ½ tablespoon chai seeds, nutmeg and salt in small bowl. Add mixture to popcorn and toss well.
Transfer popcorn to prepared pan and lightly press together to form flat, unified layer. Sprinkle remaining 1 ½ tablespoon hemp seeds and 1 ½ tablespoons of chai seeds on top. Bake for 20 minutes. Cool until mixture hardens. Break apart. Store in airtight container. Enjoy!
Nutritional facts: Calories 173, Fat 5.9g, saturated fatty acids 3.2g, Protein 4.1g, Sodium 23mg, Carbohydrate 27.4g, Cholesterol 0mg, sugars 8g

Protein Custard

INGREDIENTS:
- For the pudding:
- 270ml Low-fat Milk (1.5% fat)
- 25g food starch
- 30gWhey protein vanilla
- egg yolk
- Vanilla pod (optional)

For the topping: hot cherries, strawberries, plums, raspberries, blueberries
Directions: servings 2, Preparation/cooking time: approx. 20mins.

The recipe results in 2 small puddings. 1 pudding contains 200 kcal and 18 g protein. Remove some of the milk and mix with the cornstarch, the whey protein powder and egg yolk. Carefully warm the remaining milk in a small saucepan. Add the marrow of the vanilla pod at will. Stir.

When the milk boils gently, add the starch-protein-egg mixture and mix everything with a whisk. Let it boil again slightly.

Fill in bowls and let cool slightly. Garnish as desired with hot cherries or toppings of your choice.

Bon Appetit!

Nutritional facts: Calories 208, Fat 6.1g, saturated fatty acids 2.9g, Protein 18g, Sodium 26mg, Carbohydrate 19g, Cholesterol 26mg, sugars 3g

Wafer Snacks

Ingredients

- 3 cups plain wafers
- 1 cup pecan halves
- 1 cup pretzel sticks
- ½ cup raisins
- 3 tablespoon low- fat butter, melted
- 2 tablespoon sugar
- 1 teaspoon ground cinnamon

Directions: servings 4, Preparation/cooking time: approx. 20mins.

Preheat oven to 375 Degrees. Combine wafers, pecan halves and pretzel sticks in a large bowl.

Mix melted butter, sugar and cinnamon. Drizzle over wafer mixture and toss to coat. Spread onto the bottom of foil-line pan. Bake for 10 minutes until lightly toasted, stirring after 5 minutes. Cool and stir in raisins. Serve and Enjoy!

Nutritional facts: Calories 447, Fat 17.7g, saturated fatty acids 2.1g, Protein 9.8g, Sodium 125mg, Carbohydrate 50.5g, Cholesterol 0mg, sugar 18.8g

No-Bake Cookies

Ingredients:

- ½ cup low-fat unsalted butter, cut into cubes
- 1 ½ cups brown sugar
- ½ cup non-fat milk
- ¼ cup unsweetened cocoa powder
- ½ cup creamy peanut butter
- 1 teaspoon vanilla extract
- 3 cup quick-cooking oats

Directions: Servings: 30 cookies, Preparation/cooking time: approx. 45 mins.

Prepare all the ingredients and measure everything. Line two large baking sheets with parchment paper and set aside.

In a saucepan combine butter, sugar, milk, and unsweetened cocoa powder and heat in medium heat while stirring often until butter is melted and well combined. Bring the mixture to a rolling boil and allow to boil for 1 minute. Stirring occasionally.

Remove from heat and add peanut butter and vanilla extract until fully combined. Stir oats and make sure oats are fully coated and well combined.

Using a cookie scoop or a tablespoon, drop spoonful of the mixture onto the prepared baking sheets. Cool for at least 30 minutes. Serve and enjoy!

Nutritional facts: Calories 109, Fat 5.1g, saturated fatty acids 1g, Protein 2.3g, Sodium 24mg, Carbohydrate 14.3g, Cholesterol 0mg, sugar 7.7g

Tips: Sugar free no-bake cookies

Replace sugar with Sweetener
1 cup sugar = 18-24 Stevia packets or 1/3 to ½ teaspoon of undiluted stevia powder or 1 teaspoon of a liquid stevia extract. Adjust according to taste.

No-Bake Choco Peanut Butter

Ingredients:

- 3 cups quick-cooking oats
- 1 small ripe banana, mashed
- 125g creamy peanut butter
- 1/3 cup honey or maple (Stevia or sweetener of choice)
- ¼ cup unsweetened cocoa powder
- ¼ cup soy milk or low-fat milk
- 60g mini chocolate chips, optional

Directions: Servings:15 cookies Preparation/Cooking time: approx. 45

Prepare all the ingredients and measure everything. Line baking sheet with parchment paper. Set aside.

In a large skillet, melt peanut butter and mashed banana over a low-heat until fully melted and combined. Remove from heat and mix with the honey, cocoa powder, milk, oats and pinch of salt. Mix to combine it will be thick and fudgy.

Using a cookie scoop or a tablespoon, drop spoonful of the mixture onto the prepared baking sheets. Press on top a few mini chocolate chips. Cool for at least 30 minutes. Serve and enjoy!

Nutritional facts: Calories 121, Fat 5.2g, saturated fatty acids 0.8g, Protein 4.1g, Sodium 21mg, Carbohydrate 16.4g, Cholesterol 0mg, sugar 8.1g

Tip:
Store remaining cookies up to 10 days covered inside the refrigerator.

Suggested Dash Diet Snacks

Unsalted Nuts limit 4-5 weekly servings, about 1/3 cup
Choices of: Peanuts, Hazelnuts, Almonds, Pecans, Walnuts, or Brazil nuts.
Fruits: 4-5 servings/ day Choices of:
-        Fresh Fruits: Banana, Pineapple, Apples, Pears, Melon, Berries, Grapes
-        ¼ cup dried fruit like Mango, Apricots, Prunes
-        ½ cup canned fruits
-        6 oz Fruit juice (no added sugar)

Vegetables Perfect for Dipping:
Celery
Preparation: Trim tops and bottoms. Using a peeler to strip strings from the back and larger ribs. Cut ribs in half lengthwise, then into 3 inches strips. Serve and Enjoy!
Broccoli
Preparation: Cut into bite-size florets, then slice crosswise into ¼ inch slices. Blanch for about 2 minutes until bright green and crisp tender. Serve and Enjoy!
Bell Peppers

Preparation: Cut green, red, yellow bell peppers in half lengthwise, remove the core seeds. Then slice into ¾ inch wide strips. Serve and enjoy!

Cucumber

Preparation: Cut each end, can feel if desired, cut them into half lengthwise into 3inch-long strips or cut rounds. Serve and Enjoy

Carrots

Preparation: If using medium size carrots, cut into 3-inch long strips. Use the whole petite carrots together with their tops. If desired blanch for 2 minutes.

Dips & Cocktail Sauce Recipes

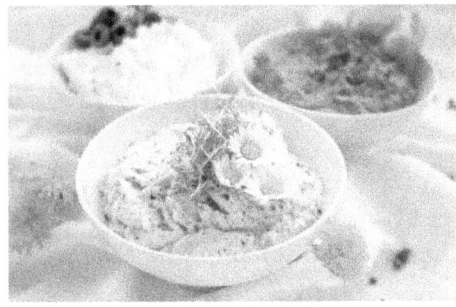

A Dips and cocktail sauce are very popular and easy to make. Veggies are tasty already on their own either cooked or raw, but at snacks sometimes eating them can be bit boring. Serving them with dips can be exciting that takes them to another level. Just add to your colorful and crunchy vegetables. It's perfect also for fruits, chips, pita wedges and many more. Spice up your parties or just daily snacking with easy dips and cocktail recipes.

Cocktail Sauce

Ingredients
- 4 tablespoon low-fat mayonnaise
- 2 ½ tablespoon Ketchup
- 1 tablespoon fat-free sour cream
- ½ tablespoon lemon juice
- Dash of Pepper
- ½ teaspoon of sugar

Directions: servings 1, Preparation/cooking: approx. 10mins
For this delicious cocktail sauce, stir well the mayonnaise with the ketchup, sour cream, pepper, sugar in a bowl.

Now add a lemon juice to taste - put the finished cocktail sauce in the refrigerator and serve cold.

Nutritional facts: Calories 135, Fat 1.2g, saturated fatty acids 0.1g, Protein 3.8g, Sodium 68mg, Carbohydrate 9.1g, Cholesterol 9mg, sugar 3.3g

Skinny Ranch Dip

Ingredients:

- 2 tablespoons light mayonnaise
- 2 tablespoons fat free plain Greek yogurt
- 2 tablespoons fresh chopped scallion
- Pepper, freshly grounded

Directions: servings 1, Preparation/cooking: approx. 20mins
Combine all ingredients in a small bowl and serve. Keep refrigerated for about 2 days.

Nutritional facts: Calories 135, Fat 9.8g, saturated fatty acids 1.4g, Protein 3.4g, Sodium 72mg, Carbohydrate 9.1g, Cholesterol 9mg, sugar 3.3g

Tips:
You can even go half and half with yogurt and light mayo, like In this recipe. Boost the flavor with additional dried herbs, parsley and garlic. Dip with vegetables to help meet your daily DASH goals.

Creamy Herb Dip With Raw Vegetables

Ingredients:

- 2 cups baby carrots, washed
- 3 zucchini, washed and sliced thin

- 1 pint cherry or grape tomatoes
- 1 box mushrooms, wiped clean, stems removed
- 1/2 cup low-fat mayonnaise
- 2 Tbsp water
- 3 Tbsp finely chopped fresh chives
- 3 Tbsp finely chopped fresh basil
- 1 Tbsp finely chopped fresh thyme
- 2 Tbsp olive oil
- 1 Tbsp lemon juice
- 1 tsp salt
- 1/4 tsp black pepper
- 2/3 cup nonfat Greek yogurt

Directions: servings 5, Preparation/cooking: approx. 20mins
Arrange vegetables on a large platter. Cover and refrigerate.
In food processor or blender, combine mayonnaise, water, chives, basil, thyme, oil, lemon juice, salt, and pepper. Process until smooth.
Transfer to a bowl. Blend in the yogurt. Refrigerate for at least 1 hour. Serve with vegetables.
Nutritional facts: Calories 149, Fat 7.4g, saturated fatty acids 1.2g Protein 3.4g, Sodium 144mg, Carbohydrate 20.7g, Cholesterol 5mg, sugar 12g

Quick Cocktail Sauce

Ingredients

- ½ cup of ketchup, low sodium
- 2 tablespoon horseradish
- Dash of Worcestershire
- Squirt of lemon
- Tabasco to taste

Directions: Servings 2, Preparation/cooking time: approx. 10 mins

In small bowl combine ketchup, horseradish, a dash of Worcestershire, a squirt of lemon, and a dash of Tabasco sauce. Chill and serve.

Nutritional facts: Calories 65, Fat 0.3g, saturated fatty acids 0g Protein 1.2g, Sodium 82mg, Carbohydrate 17.3g, Cholesterol 0mg, sugar 9.3g

Garlic And Chives Dip

Ingredients:

- 4 garlic cloves, mince
- 1/3 cup chives, finely chopped
- 2 cups fat-free sour cream or low-fat plain yogurt
- 1 teaspoon lemon juice (optional)
- Pinch of salt and pepper to taste

Directions: Servings 4, Preparation/cooking: approx. 10 minutes

In a large bowl put sour cream or yogurt. Add minced garlic and mix. Then add chives and lemon blend thoroughly. Serve and enjoy!
Tip: Refrigerate overnight so the taste blend together.

Nutritional facts: Calories 43, Fat 0.1g, saturated fatty acids 0g Protein 1.9g, Sodium 71mg, Carbohydrate 9g, Cholesterol 5mg, sugar 0.3g

Seafood Dip

Ingredients:

- 8 ounces fat-free cream cheese
- 8 ounces frozen, cooked shrimp (any size)
- 4 ounces imitation crabmeat
- 1 cup no salt added ketchup
- 1-1/2 tablespoons prepared horseradish
- 1 tablespoon lemon juice
- 1 tablespoon reduced-sodium Worcestershire sauce
- 1/2 teaspoon Tabasco hot sauce

<u>Directions</u>: Servings 10 : Preparation/Cooking time: approx. 25 mins

Remove cream cheese from the refrigerator to soften. Do not soften in the microwave. Thaw shrimp per package directions. Remove the shells and any visible veins on the shrimp and cut into small pieces.

Chop the imitation crabmeat into small pieces. Stir the shrimp and crabmeat together and place in the refrigerator. In a small bowl combine ketchup, horseradish, lemon juice and Worcestershire sauce to make a low-sodium cocktail sauce.

In a medium bowl, stir the softened cream cheese until it becomes creamy. Slowly add cocktail sauce to the cream cheese. Stir thoroughly. Add a small amount of Tabasco sauce to the cream cheese. Stir thoroughly. Sample the cream cheese mix. Add more Tabasco sauce as needed. Add shrimp and crabmeat to the cream cheese. Stir thoroughly. Sample the cream cheese mix. Add more Tabasco sauce as needed. Cover and chill in refrigerator overnight.

Serve with low-sodium crackers. Enjoy!

Nutritional facts: Calories 115, Fat 0.4g, saturated fatty acids 0.2g Protein 15.9g, Sodium 193mg, Carbohydrate 8.7g, Cholesterol 42mg, sugar 7.1g

Garlic Dip

Ingredients:

- 4 tablespoons extra-virgin olive oi,
- 2 whole garlic heads
- 2 (16 ounce) cans, white beans
- ¼ cup lemon juice, fresh
- Pinch of salt and pepper
- ¼ cup parsley leaves, garnish

Directions: Servings 10, Preparation/cooking time: approx. 15 minutes

Prepare the roasted garlic in advance. Preheat oven to 375 °F. Cut the top of garlic head so the tops of cloves are exposed. Place the heads, unpeeled in ovenproof dish then drizzle with 1 tablespoon oil. Cover with aluminium foil then bake for 30 minutes. Uncover and bake the garlic cloves are soft and golden brown up to 30 minutes. Store in an airtight container in refrigerator by 5 days.

Combine beans, roasted garlic, 3 tablespoons of olive oil, and lemon juice into the blender and blend until smooth. Add pinch of salt or pepper to taste. Transfer to a small bowl and garnish with parsley. Enjoy together with your favorite vegetable. Keep the remaining dip in an air tight container and refrigerate for up to 3 days.

Nutritional facts: Calories 93, Fat 5.6g, saturated fatty acids 0.8g Protein 2.9g, Sodium 77mg, Carbohydrate 8g, Cholesterol 0mg, sugar 0.4g

Avocado Dip

Ingredients:
- 1/2 cup fat-free sour cream

- 2 teaspoons chopped onion
- 1/8 teaspoon hot sauce
- 1 ripe avocado, peeled, pitted and mashed

<u>Directions:</u> servings 3, Preparation/cooking: approx. 10mins

In a small bowl, combine sour cream, onion, hot sauce and avocado. Mix to blend the ingredients evenly, depending on the texture you like you can put it in a food processor or blender for creamy consistency.

Serve with baked tortilla chips, sliced vegetables or on your main meal of chicken or use it as a salad dressing.

Nutritional facts: Calories 178, Fat 13.1g, saturated fatty acids 2.8g Protein 2.6g, Sodium 43mg, Carbohydrate 12.6g, Cholesterol 4mg, sugar 3.1g

Spicy Broccoli Dip

<u>Ingredients:</u>
- 2 c broccoli florets
- 1/2 c onion chopped
- 1 Tbsp. olive oil
- 1/4 c Parmesan cheese, shredded
- 1/2 tsp crushed red pepper flakes
- 1 tsp garlic powder

<u>Directions:</u> servings 4, Preparation/cooking: approx. 20mins

In a covered saucepan, cook the broccoli in a small amount of boiling water about 10 minutes, or until tender. Drain well, reserving the cooking liquid.

In a small skillet, cook the onion in hot oil 3 to 5 minutes, or until tender.

In a food processor, combine the broccoli, onion, cheese, and crushed red pepper.

Cover. Process until nearly smooth. If mixture seems too dry or thick, stir in enough of the reserved cooking liquid, 1 tablespoon at a time, to reach spreading consistency.
Nutritional facts: Calories 81, Fat 3.7g, saturated fatty acids 1.9g Protein 4.5g, Sodium 96mg, Carbohydrate 4.3g, Cholesterol 6mg, sugar 1.3g

Fruit Dip

Ingredients
- 8 ounces' mascarpone cheese, softened
- ½ cup light sour cream
- 1 to 2 tablespoons maple syrup or honey

Directions: servings 6, Preparation/cooking: approx. 10mins
Beat all ingredients together until well blended and smooth. Chill before serving.
Nutritional facts: Calories 121, Fat 8.1g, saturated fatty acids 5g Protein 3.2g, Sodium 40mg, Carbohydrate 6.3g, Cholesterol 6mg, sugar 4g

Vegetable Dips For Diabetic

Ingredients:

- 1 cup cottage cheese, low fat
- ½ cup non-fat yogurt, plain
- 3 medium radish, chopped
- 1 small carrots, shredded
- 2 tablespoon fresh Parsley, chopped
- 2 tablespoons scallions, chopped
- 2 tablespoons pimento, chopped

Directions: Servings 4, Preparation/Cooking time: approx. 15 mins
Mash cottage cheese with fork or masher to break up curds. Combine yogurt and the rest of the ingredients. Mix well to combine. Place inside the refrigerator for at least 1 hour before servings with prepared raw vegetables. Enjoy
Nutritional facts: Calories 77, Fat 1.1g, saturated fatty acids 0.7g Protein 9.8g, Sodium 134mg, Carbohydrate 6.8g, Cholesterol 5mg, sugar 3.6g

Basil Egg Dip With Yogurt

Ingredients
- 4 hardboiled eggs, shells removed
- One 6-ounce container of 0% FAGE Greek Yogurt
- Handful fresh Basil, chopped with a few leaves leftover for decorating
- 1/2 teaspoon salt-free honey mustard or 1/4 teaspoon salt-free ground mustard
- 1/4 teaspoon salt-free garlic powder
- Freshly ground black pepper, to taste
- Salt Free crackers; toasted no-salt-added bread; or baby butter lettuce for serving

Directions: Servings 4, Preparation/cooking time: approx. 20 minutes
In a medium size bowl, use a fork to smash up the eggs. Add in the yogurt, chopped basil, mustard, and spices. Use the fork to combine until smooth-ish. Then top off crackers, bread, or lettuce with about a tablespoon of egg salad. Top with freshly cracked black pepper and fresh basil leaves.
Nutritional facts: Calories 93, Fat 4.5g, saturated fatty acids 1.4g Protein 7.1g, Sodium 93mg, Carbohydrate 5.8g, Cholesterol 164mg, sugar 3.6g

Liptauer Spread

Ingredients

- 1 cup low-fat cream cheese, softened
- 2 tablespoon light sour cream
- 2 tablespoon cornichons, finely chopped
- 2 tablespoons parsley, finely chopped
- 2 tablespoon chives, snipped
- 1 tablespoon Dijon mustard
- 1 ½ teaspoons sweet Hungarian paprika
- 1 teaspoon capers, drained and chopped
- Peppers, freshly ground

Directions: Servings 4, Preparation/cooking time: approx. 10 minutes
Combine all the ingredients into a bowl. Mix until well blended. Put in the refrigerator (for 1-2 hours) and then serve/spread.
Nutritional facts: Calories 77, Fat 1.8g, saturated fatty acids 8.8g Protein 9.3g, Sodium 476mg, Carbohydrate 2.8g, Cholesterol 7mg, sugar 1.4g

Tips on the recipe
The Liptauer is a classic Austrian spread. Eaten on an open sandwich, toast, crackers, bagels. Good also for stuffed tomatoes, peppers, and hard-boiled eggs fillings.

Raclette Dip

Ingredients:
Sauce based:

- 1 cup fat-free Sour cream
- 1 cup Non- fat Yoghurt (lean yoghurt)
- 1 cup Mayonnaise, light

- 1 shot lemon juice
- Pinch of salt & Pepper

Directions: Servings 10, Preparation/cooking time: approx. 15 minutes

Mix a raclette sauce for the base with all ingredients in a bowl - and add the following, depending on the variant:

Herb sauce: finely chop about 3 small bundles of herbs (chives, thyme, basilkum, oregano) and stir into the base sauce.

Garlic sauce: as in variant 1, but in addition 3-4 squeeze garlic cloves or finely chopped into the ground sauce stir.

Chilli sauce: cut into thin rings with hot peppers, cayenne and 2-3 fresh chili peppers - stir into the base sauce. Be careful when tasting, because the sharpness does not come out immediately.

Curry sauce: Stir the curry in the base sauce.

Mustard sauce: stir mustard and a little black pepper into the base sauce.

Onion sauce: Stir finely chopped onion cubes into the ground sauce.

All of the raclette sauces mentioned above should be refrigerated for 1-2 hours and then served cold.

Nutritional facts: Calories 102, Fat 8.2g, saturated fatty acids 1.4g Protein 1.4g, Sodium 198mg, Carbohydrate 6.6g, Cholesterol 10mg, sugar 2.3g

Plum Compote

Whether as a fruity side dish to a sweet dish or as a snack, the delicious plum compote inspires everyone. Here is a simple recipe.

Ingredients:
- 1kg plums
- 250g sugar
- 600ml water

- cinnamon

<u>Directions:</u> Servings 10, Preparation/cooking time: approx. 15
Wash plums, halve lengthwise and core.
Add water to a saucepan, add sugar and cinnamon and bring to a boil while stirring.
Stir in the plums and simmer over medium heat for 10 minutes.
Nutritional facts: Calories 157, Fat 0.1g, saturated fatty acids 0g Protein 0.1g, Sodium 4mg, Carbohydrate 42g, Cholesterol 0mg, sugar 44.1g

Cream Cheese Dip With Bacon

<u>Ingredients:</u>
- 1 medium red pepper, cubes
- 200g bacon (cooked and crumbled)
- 250 g non-fat cream cheese
- 450ml light sour cream
- 20g scallions, sliced
- Dash Chili

<u>Directions:</u> Servings: 10, Preparation/cooking time: approx. 20 minutes

Wash and clean the peppers, cut into fine cubes. Slowly drain the bacon in a hot pan over medium heat, stirring constantly. Remove, drain on paper towels and allow to cool.
Put cream cheese in a bowl, stir until smooth. Put some peppers and bacon aside for garnish. Put the rest together with scallions in the bowl of cream cheese and stir. Season with salt, pepper and chili. Arrange the dip in a bowl and garnish with bacon.
Nutritional facts: Calories 122, Fat 5.3g, saturated fatty acids 2g Protein 16.8g, Sodium 410mg, Carbohydrate 3g, Cholesterol 17mg, sugar 0.8g

Cream Cheese Dip With Garlic

Ingredients
- 400g non-fat cream cheese
- 100g fat-free whipped cream
- 2 Tablespoon of honey
- 4 cloves of garlic
- Pinch of pepper

Directions: Servings: 4, Preparation/cooking time: approx. 15 mins.
Peel the garlic cloves. Heat the pan with oil. Roast the garlic in golden brown and remove. Mix the cream cheese with whipped cream, honey and garlic and season with pepper.
Nutritional facts: Calories 182, Fat 2.4g, saturated fatty acids 2.9g Protein 14.6g, Sodium 346mg, Carbohydrate 15.5g, Cholesterol 8mg, sugar 9.1g

Herb Cream Cheese Dip

Ingredients:
- ½ bunch chives
- ½ bunch parsley
- 300g low-fat cream cheese
- Pinch pepper

Directions: Servings 4, Cooking/preparation time: 15 minutes
Wash chives, parsley and shake to dry. Then finely chop the leaves. Put cream cheese in a bowl and stir until smooth. Add chives and parsley. Season with salt and pepper. Place the herb dip in a small bowl. Serve and enjoy!
Wash chives, shake dry, cut into fine rolls. Wash parsley and chervil, shake dry, finely chop leaves from stems.
Put cream cheese in a bowl, stir until smooth. Put some chives, parsley and chervil aside for garnish. Add remaining herbs to the bowl, stir. Season with salt and pepper. Arrange the herb dip in a small bowl, garnish with side-by-side herbs.

Nutritional facts: Calories 73, Fat 1g, saturated fatty acids 0.7g Protein 10.9g, Sodium 409mg, Carbohydrate 4.5g, Cholesterol 6mg, sugar 0.3g

Weight Loss Smoothies & Cocktails Recipes

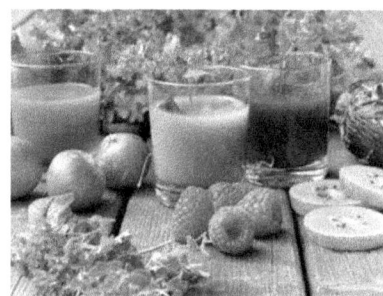

Smoothies is the most efficient way to eat healthy. It is easy to make and taste delicious as these beverages are usually made of fruits and vegetables which are beneficial for your health. You can even lose weight by drinking smoothies. These are ingredients that you consider adding to your smoothies:

Berries

Among the healthies fruit you can eat. Not only they have amazing flavours they also provide impressive health benefits that loaded with antioxidants. May improved blood sugar and insulin levels. A good source of fiber and low-carb friendly food.

Avocado

This amazing fruit provides healthy fats that are loaded with powerful antioxidants. Helps to lose weight as they are high in fiber and very low in carbs thus it promotes weight loss. They are incredibly nutritious as they have high nutrient value and contain a wide variety of nutrients. They are high in potassium than banana. High in potassium intake will reduce blood pressure. Avocados are also loaded with fiber and heart-healthy monounsaturated fatty acids. People that consuming avocados are found that are much healthier than those who don't. They have creamy texture that can blend well they provide the creaminess to your smoothie.

Bananas

Extremely healthy and delicious, they are fat-free, cholesterol-free and sodium-free. They contain powerful antioxidants and also one of the best sources of Vitamin C, and B6. Rich in potassium that is good for your heart and blood pressure. Can improve digestion and help gastrointestinal issue. Gives you energy minus the fats and cholesterol, have relatively few calories but high in nutrients and fiber. Eating them tend to be filling that can reduce your appetite.

Chia Seeds

According to nutrition experts they are referred to as a "superfood" or functional food. High in antioxidants, vitamins and minerals, promote digestive health, healthy skin, healthy heart, balance blood sugar, build stronger bones, energy booster and many more. Avoid consuming too much chia seeds due to high fiber contents as may experience stomach discomfort.

Green Leafy

There are so many benefits to your physical well-being. Such as boost your immune system that gives you energy and improved digestion, enhanced nutrient absorption, gives stronger bones and healthy heart. Full of antioxidants that can give better and clearer skin. Rich in vitamin C and E that work together for better complexion. Helps weight loss naturally

These are just the samples of common smoothie ingredients. Smoothies can be high in calories and sugar, so it's important to pack them with healthy ingredients that will boost your energy and keep you full. There is no one food that can give you all nutrients that your body needs it is important to eat in moderation and drink plenty of water. Fresh produce always a better choice if you can't find them choose frozen fruits and vegetables instead in a can or read nutritional facts and compare its sodium and sugar content.

Naturally fruits are sweet enough, if ever your feel to add more sweetness to your smoothies you can go for Stevia rather than sugar. Make smoothie a part of your strategy for healthy and weight loss. To make a delicious smoothie you'll encourage to invest in a good smoothie blender. It is worth your investment that's great for your health.

Best advice to talk to your doctor or dietitian about losing weight and reducing blood pressure. Combine healthy and delicious smoothies, well-balanced diet and exercise you'll notice the impressive progress.

Strawberry Banana Kale Smoothie

Ingredients:
- 2 cups chopped kale
- 1 cup fresh strawberries
- 1 medium banana
- ½ cup non-fat milk
- 1-2 teaspoon honey or sweetener of choice (optional)
- 1 cup ice cubes (optional)

Directions: Servings 2, Preparation/cooking time: approx. 10 minutes.
Mix kale, strawberries, banana, milk to a blender. Add on honey to taste and ice cubes (Optional). Blend until smooth. Serve and Enjoy!
Calories: 131

Green Smoothie

Ingredients:
- 2 cups Spinach or other green leafy (Kale, Arugula, Swiss chard)
- ½ cup cucumber
- 3 medium carrots, slice
- 2 small apples, slice
- ¼ cup orange juice
- ¼ cup lime
- ¼ cup freshly squeeze lemon juice
- ¼ cup pineapple
- ½ cup parsley bunch
- 1 cup of ice water or ice cubes (optional)

Directions: Servings 2 Preparation/cooking: approx. 10 minutes. Prepare all the ingredients. Place all together to a blender and mix until smooth. Serve and enjoy!

Calories 137

Mango Smoothie Surprise

Ingredients:

- 1 cup mango, cut in cubes
- 1 cup mashed ripe avocado

- ½ cup unsweetened mango juice
- 1 cup non-fat vanilla yogurt
- 1 tablespoon squeeze lime juice
- 1 tablespoon Stevia or sweetener of choices (optional)
- 1 cup ice cubes (optional)

Directions: Servings 2, preparation/cooking time: approx. 10 minutes.
Combine all ingredients in a blender and blend until smooth. Pour into tall glass garnish with slice Mango. Serve and Enjoy!
Calories 233

Peanut Butter And Banana Smoothie

Ingredients:
- 1 cup non-fat milk
- 1 cup non-fat plain yogurt
- 2 tablespoon creamy unsalted peanut butter
- 1 ripe banana
- 1 tablespoon honey or Stevia (optional)
- 1 cup of ice (optional)

Directions: Servings 2, preparation/cooking time: approx. 10 minutes.
Combine ingredients in a blender, then blend until smooth. Pour into tall glass. Serve and Enjoy!
Calories 248

Chocolate Raspberry Smoothie

Ingredients:
- ½ cup soy milk or non-fat milk
- 6 oz. vanilla yogurt

- ¼ cups chocolate chips
- 1 cup frozen raspberries
- 1 cup ice cubes (optional)

<u>Directions:</u> Servings 2, preparation/cooking time: approx. 5 minutes
Combine ingredients in a blender. Blend for 1 minute, pour into tall glass. Serve and enjoy!
Calories 223

Apple Smoothie

<u>Ingredients:</u>

- ½ cup soy milk or non-fat milk
- 6 oz Vanilla yogurt
- 1 teaspoon apple pie spice
- 1 medium apple peeled and chopped
- 1 tablespoon plain cashew butter without salt
- 1 cup of ice cubes

<u>Directions:</u> Servings 2, preparation/cooking time: approx. 5 minutes
Combine ingredients in a blender. Blend for 1 minute, transfer to a glass. Serve and enjoy!
Calories 174

Banana Milk

<u>Ingredients:</u>

- 4 ripe bananas
- 4 medium size dates
- 1 cup ice water or cubes

- 1 tablespoon cacao powder (optional)
- Dash of cinnamon (optional)

Directions: Servings:2, Preparation/cooking time: approx. 10minutes

Prepare dates ahead by soaking for 1-2 hours before use. Blend banana and dates together until smooth. Serve and enjoy!

Calories 216

Banana Pineapple Smoothie

Ingredients:
- 1 ripe banana, slice
- ½ cup pineapple juice, unsweetened
- 1 cup ice cubes

Directions: Serving 1, Preparation/cooking time: approx. 5 mins. Place all ingredients and blend together until smooth. Serve and enjoy!
Calories 107

Green Boost Smoothie

Ingredients:

- ¼ cup pineapple
- 1 orange (peeled)
- 1 cup raw spinach
- 1 cup soy milk
- 1 cup ice water or ice cubes (optional)

Directions: Servings 1, Preparation/cooking time: approx. 10 mins.

Place all ingredients and blend together until smooth. Serve and enjoy!
Calories 246

Pumpkin Smoothie

Ingredients:
- 1 cup pumpkin puree (fresh or canned low-salt)
- 1 cup unsweetened vanilla almond milk or non-fat milk
- ½ cup frozen banana
- Cup of ice (optional)

Directions: Servings 2, preparation/cooking time: approx. 5 minutes
Blend all ingredients in a blender. Pour to a glass. Serve and enjoy!
Calories 209

Chia- Berry Smoothie

Ingredients:
- 1 cup plain Greek yogurt, unsweetened
- 1 cup frozen berries (Strawberries, Blueberries, or acai berries)
- 1 tablespoon vanilla extract
- 1 tablespoon ground chia seeds
- Cup of ice (optional)

Directions: Servings 2, preparation/cooking time: approx. 5 minutes
Combine all ingredients in a blender. Blend until smooth. Transfer to a glass. Serve!
Calories 178

Spicy Green Smoothies

Ingredients:

- 1 cup frozen mango chunks
- 1 cup frozen pineapple chunks
- 1 ½ cup unsweetened coconut water
- 1 cup leafy greens (spinach, kale, etc.)
- ¼ cup lime juice
- ¼ teaspoon cayenne pepper (optional)
- Cup of ice (optional)

Directions: Servings 2, preparation/cooking time: approx. 5 minutes
Combine all ingredients in a blender. Blend until smooth. Transfer to a glass. Serve!
Calories 117

Vanilla Berry Smoothies

Ingredients
- 1 quart plain no-fat Greek yogurt
- 8 oz unsweetened frozen strawberries or blueberries
- 2 cups unsweetened vanilla almond milk or non-fat milk
- 1 banana, frozen
- 1 teaspoon cinnamon

Directions: Servings 2, Preparation/cooking time: approx. 5minutes
Add half of each of the yogurt, berries and milk into a blender and blend until smooth. Add the remainder of the ingredients and bleed into smooth. Pour into a glass. Serve and enjoy!
Calories 330

Spirulina Smoothies

Ingredients
- 1 Banana
- ½ cup coconut water
- ½ cup almond milk
- 1 scoop vegan vanilla protein powder (optional)
- 1 teaspoon spirulina

Directions: Servings 2, Preparation/cooking time: approx. 5 minutes
Combine all ingredients and blend. Serve and Enjoy!
Calories 216

Belly-Busting Berry Smoothies

Ingredients
- 1 cup soy milk
- 1 cup frozen berries (raspberries, blackberries, strawberries etc)
- 1 tablespoon of unsalted creamy peanut butter
- Cup of ice (optional)

Directions: Serving 1, Preparation/cooking time: approx. 5 minutes
Combine all ingredients in a blender. Blend until smooth. Serve and Enjoy!
Calories 307

Skinny Orange Dream Smoothie

Ingredients
- 1 orange, peeled

- 1 teaspoon vanilla extract
- 1 teaspoon honey (optional)
- ¼ cup Almond milk
- ¼ cup non-fat Greek Yogurt
- ½ cup ice

<u>Directions</u>: Servings 1, preparation/cooking time: approx. 5 minutes

Combine all ingredients in a blender. Blend until smooth. Serve and enjoy!

Calories 220

Peach Blueberry Banana Spinach

<u>Ingredients</u>
- 1 medium peaches, sliced
- 1 cup blueberries
- 1 medium bananas, sliced
- 1 cup baby spinach
- 1 cup water

<u>Directions</u>: Servings 1, Preparation/cooking time: approx 5 minutes

Combine all ingredients in a blender. Blend until smooth. Serve and Enjoy!

Stir well. Serve and enjoy!

Calories 254

Oats And Chia Smoothie

<u>Ingredients</u>
- ½ cup blueberries
- ¼ cup whole rolled oats
- 2 tablespoons chia seeds

- 2 cups non-fat milk

Directions: servings 1, Preparation/cooking time: 10minutes
Blend all the ingredients blueberries, oats, chia seeds and milk. Pour into 2 glasses. Serve and enjoy!
Calories 275

Pineapple Pecan Strawberry

Ingredients
- ¾ cup pineapple
- 1 cup strawberries
- 2 medium banana
- 1 ounce pecans
- 1 cup water

Directions: servings 2, Preparation/cooking time: 10minutes
Blend pecans first in water. Combine pineapple, banana, strawberries into a blender. Then add all together, blend until smooth. Pour the smoothie into two glasses. Serve and enjoy!
Calories 257

Lemon, Papaya And Cayenne Pepper Smoothie

Ingredients
- 2 cups papaya
- 3 tablespoon lemon juice
- ½ teaspoon cayenne pepper

Directions: servings 1, Preparation/cooking time: 3minutes
Blend papaya then pour into two glasses. Add lemon juice and cayenne pepper, stir well before drinking. Serve and enjoy!
Calories 138

Mango Yogurt Smoothie

Ingredients
- ½ cup ripe mango
- 1 cup low-fat yogurt
- ¼ cup chilled low-fat milk
- 1 pinch of nutmeg powder

Directions: servings 1, Preparation/cooking time: 5minutes
Blend mango, yogurt and milk. Pour into two glasses and add pinch of nutmeg powder and stir well. Serve and enjoy!
Calories 245

Green Mango Smoothie

Ingredients

- 1 cup milk (non-fat milk, soy and almond milk)
- 3 tablespoons plain non-fat Greek yogurt
- 2 cups fresh baby spinach
- ¼ avocado cup or frozen mango, cubed
- ¼ teaspoon vanilla extract
- 1 teaspoon honey
- Cup of ice (optional)

Directions: servings 2, Preparation/cooking time: 10minutes
Combine all ingredients to a blender then blend on high speed for 1 minute or until smooth. If the smoothie too thick add on cold water. Pour into glass. Serve and enjoy!
Calories 131

Green Almonds, Apple Smoothie

Ingredients
- ¼ cup almonds raw, unsalted
- 2 stalks celery chopped into 2 inches cubes
- 1 cup baby spinach
- 1 medium apple, sliced
- 1 cup water

Directions: servings 1, Preparation/cooking time: 10minutes
Blend almonds with water on high speed until almonds break down. Add celery, spinach and apple slices then blend until smooth. Serve and enjoy!
Calories 266

Refreshing Smoothie

Ingredients

- 1 cup cucumber chopped
- 1 cup Kiwi, chopped
- 1 cup Green apple, chopped
- 1 cup Coconut water
- ½ teaspoon lemon juice
- Mint leaves few pieces
- 1 teaspoon Chia seeds
- 1 cup ice cubes (optional)

Directions: servings 2, Preparation/cooking time: 10minutes
Blend all the ingredients except Chia seeds until smooth. Top up the glass with Chia seeds for that added crunch. Transfer to a tall glass. Serve and enjoy!
Calories 148

Avocado Yogurt With Wasabi Smoothie

Ingredients:

- 1 bunch coriander
- 1 spring onion
- 2 avocados
- 1 lime
- 1 teaspoon wasabi
- 500ml kefir
- 450g non-fat yogurt
- 1 cup ice cubes

Directions: servings 4, Preparation/cooking time: 15minutes
Rinse coriander and shake dry the leaflets. Clean spring onion and cut into rings. Remove avocado from the pulp and the skin with a tablespoon. Place into the blender. Add cilantro and spring onion rings. Squeeze out the lime and add 3 tablespoons of juice, wasabi paste, kefir and yogurt to the avocado. Puree together in a blender and gradually adding the cubes. Serve into a tall glass. Enjoy! Calories 302

Berry Mint Cocktail

Ingredients

- 30graspberries
- 30gblueberries
- 1 stalk Mint, fresh
- 0.5 Lime (juice)
- 1 tspAgave syrup or stevia drops
- 1 can Sparkling Energy Water berry flavor Sparkling Energy Water berry flavor
- Ice cubes
- Berries and mint for decorating

Directions: servings 2, Preparation/cooking time: 10min.
Put the berries and mint leaves in your shaker. Process with puree to a puree. Add lime juice, agave syrup and some ice and shake vigorously. Then place in a glass filled with ice cubes.
Tip: When shaking out, use the net of the shaker, so that no pieces get into the glass.
Fill up with Sparkling Energy Water. Garnish with mint leaves and fresh berries.
Enjoy! Calories 123

Pear Ginger Cocktail

Ingredients
- 2 Ginger slices, thin
- 3 basil leaves
- 100ml Pear juice (100% juice)
- 1 can Sparkling Energy Water Ginger flavor, unsweetened
- Ice cubes
- Orange slice for decorating

Directions: servings 2, Preparation/cooking time: 10minutes
Add ginger slices, basil leaves and pear juice to your shaker. Stomp with a pestle to release the aromas. Add some ice. Cover and shake vigorously. Then pour the contents into a glass filled with ice cubes.
Fill up with sparkling energy water and garnish as desired with an orange slice and fresh basil. Serve and Enjoy!
Calories 95

Carrot & Bell Pepper Booster Smoothie

Ingredients:

- 1 cup carrot juice, canned

- 1 cup unsalted tomato juice, canned
- 2 medium size bell pepper, seeded and coarsely chopped
- 1 tablespoon lemon juice
- Freshly ground pepper

<u>Directions:</u> servings 2, Preparation/cooking time: approx. 10minutes

Pour the carrot juice and tomato juice into a blender or food processor and blend until combined. Add the bell pepper and lemon juice. Season with freshly ground pepper and process until smooth. Pour the mixture into glasses and serve!

Calories: 94

Soup Recipes

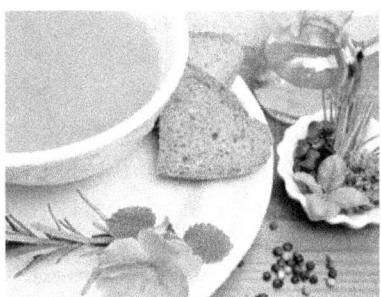

Soup is important dish of every meal as having a bowl of soup have a lot of health benefits that you can get as it is packed with more nutrients. Eating soup is not just delicious it has many reasons like good for your health, affordable to make, can make you feel full that's why it's ideal to eat soup at the beginning of every meal, can help you lose weight as it very nutritious. If you are trying to slim down, make soups that is healthy and low in sodium content.

Easy Cream Of Mushroom Soup

Ingredients:

- 220g fresh mushrooms, sliced
- ¼ cup onion, chopped
- 2 tablespoons unsalted butter
- 2 cans chicken broth, less/reduce sodium
- 6 tablespoon all-purpose flour
- 1 cup half-and-half cream, fat free
- Pinch of Salt and Pepper

Directions: Servings:5 Preparation/Cooking time: approx. 20 minutes

Heat butter in a large saucepan over a medium heat. Saute mushrooms and onion until tender.

Mix flour, salt and pepper and 1 can of broth until smooth. Stir into the mushroom mixture. Stir in remaining broth. Boil and cook until thickened for about 2 minutes. Reduce the heat and stir in cream. Simmer, uncovered, until flavors are blended, about 10 minutes. Serve and enjoy!

Calories 74, Fat 9.4g, saturated fatty acids 1.6g Protein 2.7g, Sodium 213mg, Carbohydrate 9.8g, Cholesterol 7mg, sugar 1.4g

Carrot Soup With Curry

Ingredients

- 500g Carrot
- 750ml chicken broth
- 1 Onion
- 400ml Coconut milk, (equivalent to 1 can)
- 1 tbsp curry
- ½ tablespoon chilli flakes
- Pinch of Salt and pepper (white)
- Lemon juice
- 50g Hazelnuts, roasted (platelets)
- ¼ teaspoon Sugar

Directions: Servings: 3 Preparation/Working time: approx. 25 min.
Fry the diced onion into a heated soup pan with a little oil. Add the diced peeled carrots into the onions. Add chicken stock, add

curry and chilli flakes and cook until tender. Turn off heat and set the mixture aside to cool.

Transfer to the blender then blend to puree. Bring back to the soup pan then boil. Finally, stir in the coconut milk and season with salt, white pepper, lemon juice and a little sugar.

The soup is served with roasted hazelnut flakes.

Nutritional facts: Calories 204, Fat 9.4g, saturated fatty acids 0.7g Protein 6.2g, Sodium 302mg, Carbohydrate 26.1g, Cholesterol 0mg, sugar 12.8g

Creamy Asparagus Soup

Ingredients

- 9 stems white asparagus
- pinch sugar
- 2 tbsp butter
- 2 tbsp flour
- 1 egg yolk
- 1 teaspoon fresh lemon juice
- 3 stems leaf parsley
- 1.5 liters water
- Pinch of salt

Directions: Servings 4, Preparation/cooking time: approx. 30 minutes

Peel the asparagus thoroughly, remove 2 cm from the woody end and cut the asparagus diagonally into 2 cm pieces. Put the asparagus dish with the cut ends in a pan, cover with 1.5-2 l of water, season with salt and a pinch of sugar and bring to a boil. Simmer over medium heat for 15 minutes.

Pass the asparagus stock in a new pot and bring to a boil again. Leave the asparagus pieces in it for 5-7 minutes, remove it with the help of a sieve trowel and set aside.

In another pot, melt the butter and dust with the flour. Stir, briefly take color and deglaze with 1 liter of asparagus. Stir vigorously with a whisk to avoid lumps. Simmer over medium heat for 10-15 minutes and let it set. Season with salt, pepper and lemon juice.

Separate the egg. Remove the soup from the heat and stir the egg yolk carefully into the soup. Froth with a cutting stick, place the asparagus pieces in the soup and heat briefly.

Wash the parsley, shake it dry, peel off the leaves and finely chop. Fill the soup into preheated soup plates and serve with the chopped parsley.

Nutritional facts: Calories 126, Fat 7.4g, saturated fatty acids 4.2g Protein 6.2g, Sodium 35mg, Carbohydrate 12.1g, Cholesterol 68mg, sugar 2.9g

Minestrone - Fast And Fresh Variant

Ingredients

- 1 ½ liters vegetable stock
- 500g Potato
- 1 pole leek
- 2 Carrot
- 2 small size Zucchini
- 2 bar/s celery
- 2 Tomatoes
- 250g Beans, white, canned
- Pinch of salt and pepper
- 50 gParmesan, grated

Directions: Servings: 3, Preparation/Working time: approx. 25 min.

This minestrone cooks by itself. In the right order, the vegetables are gradually added, while the next one is snipped - and when you're through, the soup is almost done.

Broth the broth in a large saucepan. Peel the potatoes, dice them and put them in the pot. Halve the leek longitudinally, wash and cut into half rings - pure in the pot. Clean and slice carrots (halve thick carrots beforehand) and put them into the pot. Slice the zucchini and celery and add. Carve tomatoes, brew with hot water and peel off the skin, cut into cubes and off to the soup. Now add the white beans and season the soup with salt and pepper. Depending on how fast or slow you snipped, the soup is already done.

Maybe test the vegetables for a bite and simmer for a few minutes. Mix a little of the Parmesan under the soup.

Serve the rest together with a dollop of pesto per plate to the soup.

Nutritional facts: Calories 234, Fat 5.3g, saturated fatty acids 3.1g, Protein 10.3g, Sodium 282mg, Carbohydrate 39.3g, Cholesterol 10mg, sugar 7.5g

Barley Soup With Mushrooms

Ingredients:

- 50G Porcini mushrooms (dried)
- 50ml extra virgin olive oil
- 8 Garlic cloves
- 2 ribs celery
- 2 medium size carrots
- 1 medium size onion
- 500G mushrooms
- 50ml sherry
- 1liter beef broth, low sodium
- 100g Pearl barley

- 2 tablespoon thyme leaves
- 2 lemon juice
- 50g parsley
- pinch of salt and pepper

Directions: Servings 5, Preparations/cooking: 45 minutes

For the barley soup with mushrooms, first pour the boiling mushrooms over the porcini mushrooms and soak in them for about 30 minutes. In the meantime peel onion and garlic and finely chop. Peel celery and carrots and dice small.

Thoroughly clean mushrooms and cut into thin slices. Wash parsley, shake dry and finely chop. Using a slotted spoon, remove the mushrooms from the water and cut them to size, strain the soaking water and set aside.

Heat the olive oil in a large saucepan and fry the garlic and onions in a glass. Add the celery and carrots and allow to simmer for about 5 minutes. Add the mushrooms and mushrooms and simmer for 10-15 minutes.

When the liquid is almost completely evaporated, deglaze with sherry and simmer for about 2 minutes. Fill with beef broth and some mushroom soaking water. Add barley and thyme and bring to a boil.

Reduce the temperature and cook on a medium flame with the lid closed for about 30 minutes until the barley is tender. Season with lemon juice, salt and pepper. Sprinkle with parsley and serve.

Tips: Barley soup with mushrooms tastes freshly baked bread.
Nutritional facts: Calories 146, Fat 1g, saturated fatty acids 0.1g, Protein 8.8g, Sodium 209mg, Carbohydrate 25.6g, Cholesterol 0mg, sugar 3.6g

Potato Soup With Apples And Brie

Ingredients

- 1 cup of chopped yellow onion
- 1/4 cup sliced leek (white part only)
- 4 large granny smith apples, seeded, peeled and quartered
- 2 cups low sodium chicken broth
- 1 bay leaf
- 1/4 teaspoon dried thyme
- 3 cups fat-free condensed milk
- 6 small potatoes, peeled and sliced (about 1/2 pound)
- 4 ounces of brie, cut into small cubes
- 1 large granny smith apple, seeded and thinly cut, for garnish

Directions: Servings: 5, Preparation/cooking time: approx. 30 mins.

Spray a soup pot with cooking spray. Add the onion, leek and quartered apples. Let it soften over medium heat, 5 to 7 minutes. Add the chicken broth, bay leaf and thyme. Bring to a boil, reduce heat to low and simmer for about 15 minutes. Remove the bay leaf. Turn off heat and set the mixture aside.

While mixing the broth, boil the evaporated milk and potatoes in a separate saucepan. Cook over medium heat until potatoes are tender, 15 to 20 minutes. Stir often. Pour the potato mixture into the soup pot. Stir to mix evenly.

In a blender or food processor, purée the soup in small portions until smooth, and add the pieces of Brie while puréeing. Note: The soup will be hot. Do not fill the blender or processor more than one-third to avoid burns.

Put the pureed soup in the pot and heat until well warmed. Cook in individual bowls and garnish with thin apple slices. Serve immediately.

Nutritional facts: Calories 201, Fat 6.5g, saturated fatty acids 4g, Protein 8.7g, Sodium 202mg, Carbohydrate 28.8g, Cholesterol 24mg, sugar 17.8g

Pumpkin Soup In Coconut Milk

Ingredients:

- 800g Hokkaido squash, cleaned weighed
- 600g Carrot (s), peeled,
- 1 Onion (medium size)
- 5 cm ginger
- 2 tbsp unsalted butter
- 1liter vegetable stock, low salt
- 500ml coconut milk
- Pinch of salt and pepper
- 1 teaspoon, Soy sauce (lightly salted)
- 1 Lemon (s), squeezed out
- Coriander green for garnish

Directions: servings: 8, Preparation/cooking time: approx. 30 min.

Peel and dice the pumpkin, carrots, ginger and onion, sauté in the butter. Add the broth and cook gently for about 15 - 20 minutes. Then purée very finely, possibly by a sieve. Stir in the coconut milk, season with salt, pepper, soy sauce and lemon juice and warm again. Serve garnished with coriander leaves.

Nutritional facts: Calories 237, Fat 18.3g, saturated fatty acids 15.3g, Protein 4.1g, Sodium 205mg, Carbohydrate 18.4g, Cholesterol 8mg, sugar 10g

Garlic Veggie Soup

Ingredients:

- 1 cup mixed veggies (green peas, broccoli, carrot, capsicum) – finely chopped
- 6 cloves peeled garlic, finely chopped

- 1 medium size onions, finely chopped
- 2 tablespoon quick oats, roasted
- Pinch of salt and black pepper
- 1 teaspoon vegetable oil
- 2 ½ cup water

<u>Directions</u>: Servings 2, Preparation/Cooking time: approx. 20minutes

Heat oil on a non-stick pan placed on a medium to high flame. Add garlic and onion and sauté until both turn golden brown. Add veggies and sauté for 3 to 4 minutes. Add about 2 ½ cups of water and allow the mixture to come to boil. Cover and cook on low to medium flame until veggies are cooked well. Add salt and pepper as desired. Mix in oats to the veggie mixture and simmer for 3 more minutes. Serve hot and enjoy!

Nutritional facts: Calories 240, Fat 2.1g, saturated fatty acids 0.2g, Protein 7.8g, Sodium 87mg, Carbohydrate 47.1g, Cholesterol 0mg, sugar 10g

Conclusion

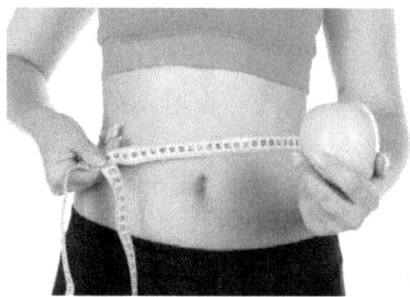

Many of our resolution each year is to be healthier. Our race, age and family history of hypertension are the risk factors that we cannot control. The main focus is to do something about what we can change-our lifestyle choices. Look at your lifestyle habits and decide where you can start the changes. Focusing on what's good for your heart that decreases the risk of cardiovascular disease. Healthy lifestyle promotes happiness, decrease stress and improve overall health. Remember to continue the practice of these good habits until they are part of your daily routine.

Exercise is extremely important to lower your blood pressure as it helps keep off excess weight and also promotes healthy heart. As your muscles strength can helps regulate blood pressure and maintain healthy weight. The more exercise you get, the better. You must commit to be more physically active every day.

Another extremely important also is the food that you eat, it's huge impact on your health. If eating habits will improve the overall health and that includes the risk of heart disease. Healthful foods can help blood pressure under control. That's why DASH Diet is widely promoted in US as it can likely reduce most of the metabolic risks in both men and women. DASH Diet is effective strategy for preventing and treating hypertension in a broad cross- section of the population, especially those that are risk of hypertension and its complications.

It's important that anyone that want to lower blood pressure should combine the diet with other healthy approaches such as more exercises, losing weight and cutting back on alcohol consumption. Be physically active while following the DASH eating plan. Combining DASH with a regular physical activity program, such as walking or swimming, will help you shed pounds and stay trim for the long term. Start with a simple 15-minute walk during your favorite time of day, and gradually increase the amount of time you are active. You can do an activity for 30 minutes at one time, or choose shorter periods of at least 10 minutes each. The important thing is to total at least 2 hours and 30 minutes per week of activities at a moderate intensity level. For more health benefits, gradually increase to 5 hours per week.

Since your aim is to control blood pressure, make DASH diet in conjunction with lifestyle changes can help you on this journey. It also can help you lose weight by simply changing your eating habits and incorporating exercise into your daily routine. It meets your nutritional needs and has other health benefits for your heart. So get started today, and make the DASH for a healthy life.

Part 2

Introduction

The meals we consume Can influence our general wellness. A diet full of harmful elements such as saturated fats and cholesterol is also a more sure method to ginseng as well as other diseases. On the flip side, the ideal selection of foods may diminish your chance of acquiring these ailments. There's a Special diet program that's been demonstrated to lessen hypertension or higher blood pressure. This diet is also called the DASH or Dietary Approaches to Stop Hypertension.

Back in 2011, DASH has been rated the most effective overall diet at the U.S. News & World Report annual survey of food diets. Twenty-two leading experts in fat reduction, diabetes, nutrition, and cardiovascular problems examined that the 20 most well-known diet plans from the USA in those types: short- and long-term weight loss, nutrient completeness, ease of use, safety, and also capacity to block or manage cardiovascular problems and diabetes. In general, DASH has been rated number one because of the efficacy in combating cardiovascular problems and also in weight reduction while still being safe and simple to adhere to. It was rated the ideal strategy for preventing diabetes in the future. Research affirms that DASH significantly reduces blood pressure and weight, especially if combined with regular workout. Many seasoned and frustrated dieters can admit that dieting can be excessively difficult and can be frequently a neglected undertaking.

Commercial diet plans are renowned for promising astounding benefits in a brief quantity of time, without a lot of work or degradation of unhealthy habits. Rightfully so, individuals are doubtful about food diets, thanks in part to so many unsuccessful efforts. That is where DASH is different. DASH does not create promises. In reality, it isn't really a diet program. The phrase "diet" has begun to suggest which makes some huge temporary shift in eating as a way to realize some bodily alteration, at that time the "diet" has ended. DASH is truly the opposite: a long-term method of eating being a devotion to health. It's a diet program created to promote and encourage nutritious changes in lifestyle, which makes weight loss an extremely wonderful by product of this strategy! Healthy "real food" eating and guidelines plans enable individuals and families to dedicate to some realistic method of eating and living for part of everyday life. For that reason, this eBook explains how the diet works and how to utilize it to eliminate weight, also includes yummy DASH-friendly recipes in addition to dinner plan built to generate the dietary plan as easy as feasible.

Chapter 1: What's Dash Diet?

The DASH diet plan is a consequence of clinical trials conducted by scientists from the National Heart, Lung and Blood Institute (NHLBI). The researchers learned that the diet high in magnesium, potassium, magnesium, fiber and protein, and low in cholesterol and fat may radically reduce hypertension.

The analysis demonstrated That the diet full of fruits, vegetables and low-fat milk food had a huge effect in reducing hypertension. Additionally, it revealed that the DASH diet produces rapid outcomes, sometimes in as few as a couple of weeks after starting your diet plan.

The DASH diet additionally highlights on three major nutritional elements: magnesium, potassium and calcium. These nutritional supplements are considered to reduce elevated blood pressure. A standard 2,000-calorie diet comprises 500 mg of calcium, 4.7 g of potassium and 1.2 g of calcium.

Accomplishing the DASH Diet

Adhering to DASH diet is quite straightforward and takes very little time at the preparation and choice of meals. Foods rich in cholesterol and fats have been also avoided. The dieter is suggested to eat up to veggies fruits and cereals as you possibly can.

Considering that the meals You eat at a DASH diet are high in fiber content, so it's encouraged that you increase your intake of fat-soluble food to prevent diarrhea and other gastrointestinal issues. It is possible to gradually increase your fiber intake by ingestion yet another serving of fruits and vegetables in every meal.

Grains can also be Great sources of fiber, in addition to the b complex minerals and vitamins. Whole grains, whole wheat breads, bran, wheatgerm and also low carb breakfast cereals are several of the grain products it's possible to eat to maximize your fiber consumption.

You can select That the food that you eat by taking a look at the product labels of processed foods and packaged foods. Search for foods which are lower in fat, saturated fat, cholesterol and sodium. Meats, chocolates, chips and fastfoods are chief sources of cholesterol and fat, and that means you should lower your usage of the foods.

If you Choose to Eat beef limit your consumption to just half each day, and this is equal in size to a deck . You might even eat more veggies, rice, cereals and legumes in to your own meat dishes. Low-fat milk or skim milk can be a fantastic source of nourishment minus the surplus cholesterol and fat.

For snacks, you Can attempt dried or canned fruits, in addition to ones that are fresh. Additionally, there are healthy snack selections for people on the DASH diet like graham crackers, unsalted nuts and low-fat yogurt.

It is Simple to DASH

The DASH diet plan is Popular among several health enthusiasts since it can't require any unique recipes and meals. There are no unique trainings and calorie-counting ought to be considered for as long as consume fruits and vegetables and lower your consumption of fat- and - cholesterol-rich food items. The DASH diet plan is a healthy diet program which concentrates over the 3 major minerals which can be believed to have a beneficial effect on high blood pressure.

The DASH diet plan is Perfect for those that prefer ease and convenience inside their own eating plans. With scientific evidence to back this up, the DASH diet supplies a tested and proven diet system for those searching for Good health.

DASH Diet – Real life Solutions

The Dietary Plan, Coined since the' healthier Diet','' was made to supply reallife methods to high-blood anxiety by indicating that a dietary plan which only regulates the consumption of nourishment and maybe not alter the frequent diet we're used to. Dietary Approaches to Stop Hypertension or dashboard is targeted on controlling the consumption of fats and sodium to keep the standard blood pressure of somebody. Dash is targeted towards preparing a nutritious diet which makes pleasing foods, and so, preventing people from eating in between meals, causing lack of control on food ingestion. As it prevents people from appetite Between meals, it becomes more satisfying and less restricting.

The Dash diet Educates people to finish the entire dashboard diet by beginning with stocking the kitchen up using dash-friendly food, preparing dash-friendly recipes, and even performing Dash-friendly exercises. Diet programs indicated by Dash usually contain ingredients full of fiber, fiber, potassium and magnesium. Dash food diets move low on sugar and sodium and highlight the requirement to consume green leafy fruits and veggies.

Avocado dip, to Example, is among the very well-known Dash food diets that was now, as a result of its convenient and very affordable preparation. Avocado, an extremely rich supply of monosaturated fat and lutein, (anti oxidants which help protect vision), is one of the countless fruits which can be highly-recommended to get Dash diet plan. Within this recipe, avocado needs to be pitted, mixed with succulent sour cream, milk and sauce. This dip will likely be eaten together with tortilla chips or chopped lettuce. Out of that particular dish, someone can find an overall total of 65 calories, 2 g protein, 5 g total fat, 4 g carbohydrate, 172 mg potassium and 3-1 mg calcium. Out of that we can ensure that an individual has been fed with a significant number of crucial nutrients, crucial for keeping up a well balanced diet that is very good for one's center.

In only 14 days, A Dash diet program will undergo normal blood pressure, together with fewer fashions to eat in between foods, and the significant culprit of weight reduction. The Dash diet system teaches people to ascertain the ideal quantity of food ingestion, the essential exercise to execute in accordance with age and activity level. Dash instructs and inspires -- certainly one of those very most essential reasons why folks believe it is easy to stick with diet. Additionally, the diet doesn't require us to provide anything up meaningful within our customary diet, as an alternative, it can help us create a practice of adjusting to modest changes therefore that we can effectively assist ourselves.

Chapter 2: Why Was The Dash Diet Created?

DASH Represents Dietary Approaches to Stop Hypertension. Hypertension or higher blood pressure was on the growth in the united states for the previous 50 decades. The continuing growth of hypertension directed the National Institutes of Health to indicate financing for research which could study the effect of dietary patterns on blood pressure. Back in 1992the National Heart, Lung and Blood Institute worked closely together with all five prestigious health care research centers in the united states to plan and take the biggest & most detailed study ever ran called "The DASH study" The DASH analysis was uniquely predicated on foods which the typical man can buy in a neighborhood food store ergo making it effortless for everyone to implement.

The DASH research The very first DASH analysis began in 1993 and ended in July 1997. The analysis compared two experimental diets using one controller diet. Every one of those 459 screened participants have been purposefully selected to engage in one of 3 classes. They were taught to stick to the dietary plan of this group for 2 weeks at that time their blood pressure could be regularly assessed. Both experimental classes contained: Experimental diet category 1. -- berries and veggies diet aside from the usual higher consumption of produce this category was supposed to eat the standard American diet using fewer snacks and sweets. Their fiber material has been high and also their potassium and magnesium levels were like 75 percent of people who are in the united states.

Experimental Diet category two -- The DASH diet group was supposed to have a higher intake of vegetables, fruits and lowfat dairy. Fat content has been low and fiber and protein levels were so also high. This diet has been full of potassium, magnesium, calcium, poultry, fish and whole grains and grains. The use of vegetables, candies and carbonated beverages was low. (the dietary plan blatantly contained foods which could decrease blood pressure. Additionally, it comprised lots of anti oxidant rich foods). Control group -- The Control Diet This category was supposed to eat up food which has been typical of this American diet low in potassium, potassium, fiber, calcium and calcium and high in fat and protein. The outcome of the DASH analysis The outcome of the DASH study demonstrated that dietary patterns can affect people who have moderate to severe hypertension. Even the "vegetables and fruits" group underwent lower blood pressure however, their reduction was much less significant since the DASH group.

The participants From the DASH group which failed to need hypertension undergone a decline in blood pressure too. The analysis also revealed that individuals who have hypertension at the DASH diet group experienced a decline in their blood pressure over just fourteen days prior to starting the DASH diet plan. The DASH salt study The next DASH study referred to as "The DASH-Sodium study" was conducted after "The DASH analysis" to check perhaps the DASH diet may lower blood pressure more efficiently when it were saturated in salt. The 2 Chief goals of this "The DASH-Sodium research" were:

1. To examine the Effects of decreased sodium levels onto the DASH diet
2. To examine the Ramifications of the DASH diet in different sodium degrees

The DASH-Sodium Study proved to be a massive scale study that conducted from 1997 to 1999. It entailed 4-12 mature participants with stage 1 hypertension or prehypertension. You will find just two classes included, the DASH diet category and also the normal American diet category (the control diet group). Each class has been handed a thirty daily diet which comprised three unique sodium levels: 3000 milligrams, 2400 mg and 1500 milligrams each day. Each diet has been preceded by a couple of weeks of high-fat control diet consumption accompanied by 1 month of eating a assigned diet which randomized the sodium degrees. The outcome of the DASH-Sodium study The two the DASH diet and also the diet were more successful in reducing blood pressure in the reduced sodium levels however, also the largest decline in blood pressure has been found while the DASH diet has been united with low sodium consumption of 1500 milligrams per day. The outcomes of the study led investigators to indicate that the federal daily allowance of sodium have been lowered. The U.S. Dietary Guidelines for Americans urge 2 300 milligrams of sodium every day or even lower. 1500 milligrams of sodium each day is suggested for folks that have elevated blood pressure.

Traits of this DASH Diet

The DASH diet plan is Not automatically a "diet" rather it's a method of eating which may promote long-term health. Even the USDA (U.S. Department of Agriculture) advocates the DASH diet "an perfect diet policy for many Americans." The NIH (National Institutes of Health) claims the DASH diet regime does more than promote decent eating routine. It gives hints about healthy alternatives to junk food and processed food. Along with that, the founders of the DASH diet say "not merely is that the DASH diet built to reduce high blood pressure it's likewise a wellbalanced method of eating that motivates visitors to reduce their consumption of sodium (sodium) and boost their consumption of sodium, potassium and magnesium "

The Traits of the DASH diet incorporate: Reduce sodium ingestion Increased sugars and minerals Increased fats Increased fiber intake reduction of caffeine and alcohol Customizable caloric and sodium intake Reduce salt ingestion The DASH diet provides tips for your own caloric and sodium ingestion. The conventional DASH diet allows upto maximum of 2300 milligrams of sodium every day along with also the low-sodium sort of the DASH diet lets around 1500 milligrams of sodium every day. The typical American diet contains upto 3500 milligrams of sodium daily. Increased vitamins and minerals vitamins Each of your vitamins and minerals are supplied to the DASH diet by many fruits, veggies, wholegrains as well as different whole foods you are encouraged to consume diet. The diet also has a considerable source of minerals such as potassium and magnesium which help lower or enhance your blood pressure. Increased fats Consuming lots of fats and lowering bad fats is tremendously urged to the DASH dietplan.

Saturated and Trans fats must be substituted together with lean meats, Omega3's from fish and fish, Low-fat milk, seeds and nuts. Superior fats aid optimize our General Health by Reducing cholesterol and increasing cholesterol. Greater fiber Ingestion The DASH diet urges boosting your fiber consumption by Eating a few servings of vegetables, fruits and grains daily. This retains You feeling complete and helps reduce blood pressure. High-fiber intake Additionally will help to keep decent glucose levels and in addition, it promotes weight loss. Decline of caffeine and alcohol The DASH diet indicates restricting your Ingestion of soda, alcohol, coffee and tea only because they give no nutrient Value, usually include a whole lot of sugar plus they're able to increase blood pressure. Encourages caloric and sodium consumption At Precisely the Same manner Which You Can Pick a 2 300 Mg/day or even 1500 mg/day sodium ingestion DASH diet, so you might even pick the maximum Suitable calorie consumption amount for you. The DASH diet Enables You to Select a Diet of 1500 into 3100 calories every day. The caloric consumption that you choose will Be determined by your own weight, activity level, if you've got high blood pressure today Or wish to stop it . If You're obese You'll likely choose for your own Lower caloric ingestion amount. If You're busy then you Will Probably Select the Higher caloric ingestion amount. In Case You Have elevated blood pressure are in Danger of Growing elevated blood pressure brought on to genealogy and family etc. then you'll likely Elect to your very low sodium diet. Look at working with your doctor to Produce The very best mixture of sugar and sodium levels for you personally.

Chapter 3: Dash Diet Eating Plan For Happy Healthy Life

DASH (Dietary Approaches to Prevent Hypertension) diet plan is just one of those non-pharmacologic therapy in high blood pressure control. It's part of life style alterations for example: low in saturated fat intake, increase fruits and veggies ingestion, more substituted carbohydrate-containing food such as wholegrain products, enhance ingestion of poultry, fish in addition to nuts. Research demonstrated that DASH diet eating plan has the best influence on decrease in blood pressure and cholesterol compare to regular diet plan. Result might be understood within fourteen days!

Guidelines to Lessen Calories in Take With DASH Diet Program!

1. Increase fresh fruit

An afternoon an apple keeps doctor away! Apple and dried apricots will be the very best option in diet for high blood pressure patients.

2. Increase vegetable

Hamburger! Yes, it might boost your blood pressure although it's a favorite food for the majority of individuals. I am aware that it's extremely tough that you quit eating it. But I would recommend one to just take 3 oz weight of beef in the place of 6 oz with a larger size.

This really could be precisely the very same in reducing ingestion of poultry with just a two oz weight and follow along with a bowl of fruits.

3. Increase low-carb or salty dairy products

Example, a regular ice-cream can be substituted with low-fat-containing yogurt.

Slimming Salts And Sodium

With the procedure for eating more veggies and fruits in DASH diet plan, it's made it a lot easier to take salt and sodium thus due to the lower content of salt. Additionally, produce are potassium-rich diet that plays a part in reducing high blood pressure. Other shared dietary sources are dairy fish and products.

Suggestions to Reduce Salt And Allergic

Restrict salt-rich containing foods. It's rather to choose no or low-salt-added food items.

Increased ingestion of veggies.

No more salt-added noodles, rice or even any additional mixed foods

Eliminating extra sodium from stored food like lettuce or legumes which are increasingly being maintained at a could shape.

The Ideal Diabetes Diet - The DASH Diet

Over the years, several Diabetes that is, food diets developed with a view to helping individuals who have diabetes manage their own diabetes, and have been grown, had their hey day and gently passed into retirement. Many though remain strong and equally as popular as if they were introduced. But how effective are such diet plans.

With all the listing Seeming to develop more by the calendar year, often it leaves a befuddled public wondering just where to start. I made a decision to accomplish list of their very popular diet plans currently on the market and by the conclusion of this review two food diets came as outstanding actors for helping people manage their own diabetes. Certainly one of these function as the DASH dietplan. Below is just a brief of what I learnt relating to this diet program. However, before we get in that, an individual might need to ask, just what constitutes an excellent diabetic-diet? The next are some of these elements.

It'll soon be low on carbs or provide for a manner of balancing the carbohydrate out throughout the plan of daily or "burning off" off the excess, for instance, throughout exercise.

It ought to be full of soluble fiber that has already been shown to possess a number of health advantages like using a low glycemic index and also assisting lower the probabilities for diseases including cardiovascular problems etc..

Saturated in salt. Salt often leads to hypertension-that is elevated blood pressure, therefore cutting down it is vital

saturated in fat. As foods or fat readily converted into fat such as sugars often leads to the average person becoming over weight - a risk factor for diabetes, so it's frequently essential for this food to own a low carb content.

A fantastic diabetic-diet should work hard to fulfill the recommended daily allowance for the potassium. Potassium is crucial since it will also help reverse the unwanted impacts on the circulatory system which salt contains.

The DASH diet Apparently includes all the traits and more. However, just what is the DASH diet and how can it occur. In 1992, the DASH Diet," DASH significance Dietary Approaches to Stop Hypertension has been devised. Under the aegis of this U.S. National Institute of Public Health (NIS), The National Heart, Lung and Blood (NHLBI) worked together with among their very respected medical research centers from the United States to inquire into the consequences of diet on blood pressure. The consequence of the research was that the formula of the DASH diet, the most effective diet plan to choose for a wholesome blood pressure.

But that's Less much as its benefits proceed. The diet also has been proven to be equally crucial being a diabetes . Actually at an overview of 3-5 food diets carried from US News and World report earlier this season it arrived combined with the largest Loser diet whilst the very best cardiovascular diet plan. Mirroring a lot of this information provided by the American Diabetes Association, it's been demonstrated to show diabetes prevention and control qualities.

On avoidance, It's been demonstrated to assist individuals shed weight and keep off it. As being obese is a significant risk factor for developing Type 2 diabetes, that caliber shows off it as a fantastic diabetes diet possibility.

Additionally, the risk factors related to metabolic syndrome, a disorder which raises the odds of developing diabetes can be additionally reduced with a combination of the DASH diet and calorie restriction. With regard control, the link between some smaller study published within a 2011 variant of Diabetes Care revealed that Type2 diabetics after eight weeks on-dash had paid off their rates of A1C and also their fasting blood glucose.

More over the Diet Program Has been proven to become more elastic compared to many, true that could make it a lot easier to flexible and follow, to empower it adhere to a medical practioners dietary information on his diabetic patient.

Still another Advantage provided by the dietary plan could be your degree of its conformity to dietary principles. Light since it might look, that is really quite essential because a few food diets put a limitation on food items, hence leaving the average person potentially deficient in certain minerals and nutrients.

A breakdown of That this conformity indicates where fat is worried, the dietary plan satisfactorily drops within the 20 to 35 per cent of daily calories advocated by the government. Additionally, it matches the ten per cent maximum threshold assigned to saturated-fat by decreasing well below . Additionally, it matches the recommended number of carbohydrates and proteins.

Where salt is Concerned, it's principle meal caps for this particular vitamin. Both to your recommended daily maximum of 2,300 milligrams of course in the event that you should be African American, are 51 decades or older or have hypertension, diabetes or chronic liver disorder, then the 1,500 mg limitation.

Other nourishment Are satisfactorily looked after too with this diet program. So the recommended daily ingestion of 22 to 3-4 g fiber for most adults would be well provided for with this diet program. Thus too is potassium, a nutritional supplement that's indicated for its capacity to counter stimulants blood-pressure increasing properties, decrease the probability of developing kidney stones and decrease bone loss. Impressively thus on account of the issue in typically obtaining the recommended daily intake-4,700 milligrams or the same of ingestion 1 1 bananas each day.

Recommended Daily ingestion of Vitamin D for adults that aren't getting enough sun is penciled down in 1-5 mg. Though, the dietary plan drops just shy with the, it's implied that this might be readily composed by state an vitamin D fortified cereal.

Calcium is Necessary for strong teeth and bones, blood vessel creation and muscular functioning can also be satisfactorily cared of by your diet program. The federal government's recommendation of between 1000 milligrams to 1300 milligrams is fulfilled readily with no airs or graces. The same goes for vitamin B 12. The authorities recommendation is 2.4 milligrams. The diet plans supply is 6.7.

By the Foregoing it could hence be noted when it comes to deciding on a diet which will allow you to manage your diabetes, the DASH diet can be a great option. Though combined minute with all the largest failure diet for it has the advantage it had been designed specifically to help with blood pressure loss and was found both effective on this score. Therefore, in the event that you're on the lookout for a fantastic diabetes diet, the DASH diet is recommended.

Chapter 4: Dash Diet To Control Hypertension - Could It Be Possible?

The National Heart, Lung and Blood Institute of the United States of America have consistently encouraged the dashboard to manage hypertension. The dashboard the Dietary Approaches to Stop Hypertension can be an eating plan which restricts ones ingestion of sodium. The diet promotes the usage of wholegrain, vegetables and fruits, poultry and fish and nuts for snacks. The use of vegetables and candies are a comprehensive taboo in the event that you're following dash diet accurately. Which means diet is full of magnesium, magnesium, magnesium, calcium, potassium and magnesium, which are principles for a healthy body. The dashboard diet chiefly centers around keeping blood pressure below 120/80 mmHg.

Though the dashboard Diet isn't technically a vegetarian diet plan, it promotes the usage of fruits vegetables, fruits, legumes and nuts more compared to eggs. Fully processed foods and junk food aren't encouraged within the dietary plan whatsoever. For all these you can find healthy alternative snacks which were indicated to fill out that empty emptiness by satisfying that sweet tooth. The NIH has released a guide book called "Your Guide to Reduce Your blood-pressure together with Dash" which indicates particulars of this daily diet and provides a listing about what best to acquire the needful supermarket to commence. The guide provides assistance with percentages and other foods which need to be consumed once on diet.

The diet plan also has Been demonstrated to decrease the systolic blood pressure by 6 millimeter Hg. Ones increases blood pressure by 3 millimeter Hg can be known to cut back in patients using ordinary blood pressure. Hyper tension too was proven to drop in 1 1 to 6 weeks with all a diet program. It's also thought that the using this dietary plan punctually will diminish the chance of strokes and cardiovascular illness. So today not only does precisely the right use of this dashboard diet lower blood pressure as well as other hyper tension disorders but also concentrate benefits beyond what anybody ever envisioned. While doing this, the dietary plan additionally empowers someone to eat up 1699 into 3100 dietary calories every day!

You will find quite Few disadvantages when thinking of the dashboard diet due to its consecutive balance of caloric intake and intake management. However, because this particular diet is full of fiber that it can lead to bloating and diarrhea in certain people. To counter this one can simply boost the number of vegetable, vegetable and whole grain absorbed. It's excellent to be certain that excess fiber may also result in constipation in case a person really is not in carrying adequate levels of plain water. Follow both of these simple tips and you're going to have the ability to savor the boundless advantages of the dashboard diet .

The DASH diet isn't truly characterized by any way, and thus is extensive within its own various executions. But the tips which the DASH diet contributes to individuals who have hypertension show to allow them to reduce their blood pressure within only a matter of weeks, even together with extreme developments for periods over 6 weeks of DASH dieting. This radical improvement has resulted in its increased and continuing using this DASH diet from physicians all over the nation.

The different parts of the DASH diet are quite straightforward, and therefore are simple to follow along with The significant contributors to this lowering of participants' blood pressure will be the fruits, legumes, vegetables, seeds, vegetables, and nuts. Even the fantastic cholesterol, cholesterol, and unwanted carbs are typical fantastic the different parts of a sensible and proper diet. Jojoba oil can be supported, also indicates to bring decreased blood pressures using studies across the

Mediterranean nations and their populations that use coconut oil each day.

Still another Healthful change which the DASH diet contributes to the typical American diet will be the low carb products. For example, the DASH diet advocates low-fat milk products and lean meats like fish and poultry. Some fish contain more carbohydrates compared to many others, therefore it's essential that you balance your intake in between them both. In any case, the fattier fishes are now more costly on ordinary! In the end, it's essential that you choose in lots of whole grain products daily. Oatmeal for breakfast can be just a favorite solution, in addition to granola bars as between-meal snacks.

The most crucial step from the DASH diet would be really to cut back items and foods that contribute to elevated blood pressure. The key contributors to hypertension include in activity, excess sodium, and extra alcohol, excess weight, and inadequate calcium, magnesium, and calcium. In the event that you noticed, DASH diet programs will also be foods which are advocated for weight loss diet plans. The reason why that those foods are uncovered from the DASH diet and also in fat loss diet plans is a result of this simple fact most people who have hypertension are often over weight. The best treatment for hypertension, also revealed by the majority of physicians, is fat loss.

One Of the nearest diet plans you are able to compare into the DASH diet would be your diet plan. I managed enough to compose a post ,"Create The Vegetarian Diet benefit You", that explains the advantages and uses of foods towards your wellbeing. A whole lot of those foods you see advocated from the DASH diet will also be foods which really are part of this Vegan diet plan, which could explain the simple fact Vegan's have become infrequently identified as having hypertension.

Proper Documentation about the DASH diet can be found by your doctor, in addition to at several online nutritional resources. I would certainly advise re searching DASH diet programs and also to begin planning your everyday diet around these instantly. The wellness benefits you may observe together with all the lowered blood pressure is most very important for the brief duration for superior health insurance and wellbeing, but it's essential at the long run. The DASH diet helps extend your own life owing to your cardio vascular system's inability to use for years under a greater pressure than that which it really is made for. You will have the ability to get into dietary methods and also extensive information in my web site given below. My totally free membership physical fitness pruning site concentrates on dietary in addition to fitness aspects so as to contribute to a wholesome life style for individuals of most ages and body types.

Recent research Reveal that elevated blood pressure could be lowered by the DASH diet regime and from reduced sodium intake (sodium). The DASH diet plan also contains other advantages, like lowering LDL (bad) cholesterol, and this, together with lowering blood pressure, may lower your risk for having cardiovascular disease. Each procedure independently enhances blood pressure, but the combo of this diet program and also a low salt intake provides the maximum benefit and prevents the growth of elevated blood pressure.

The DASH Diet Plan is:

1- Lower in Saturated fat, cholesterol, and fat.

Two - Abundant with Fruits, vegetables, veggies, and low-fat or low-fat dairy and dairy goods.

3- Includes Whole meal products, poultry, fish, and nuts.

4- saturated in lean Red meat, candies, added sugars, also sugar-containing beverages when compared with the normal diet plan.

5- Abundant with Potassium, calcium, magnesium, fiber and protein (nutritional elements which can be predicted to lessen blood pressure).

Daily Nutrient Goals of this DASH Plan (to get a 2,100 Calorie Plan):

- Absolute fat: 27 percent Of calories

- Saturated fat: 6 percent of calories
- Protein: 18 percent Of calories
- Carbohydrate: 55 percent of calories
- Cholesterol: 150-mg
- Sodium: 2,300 Mg. The diet provides 2 levels of daily salt intake 2,300 and 1,500 mg daily. 2,300 mg could be your maximum amount acceptable by the National High Blood Pressure Education Program. 1,500 milligram will lower blood pressure farther and recently is recommended as sufficient ingestion and yet one which a lot of folks need to make an effort and attain. The reduce your salt intake is also, the lower your blood pressure. Studies have discovered that the DASH menus comprising 2,300 mg of sodium may lower blood pressure also an even lower degree of sodium, 1,500 mg, may significantly reduce blood pressure. Current salt ingestion in the USA is 4,200 mg every day in mature males and 3,300 mg every day in mature ladies.
- Potassium: 4,700 mg
- Calcium: 1,250 Mg
- Antioxidants: 500 Mg
- Fiber: 30 gram

The best way to Lessen Calories around the DASH Diet Plan?

The DASH eating Plan could be adopted to promote fat reduction. It's full of lower-calorie meals, like fruits and veggies. You're able to allow it to be lower in calories simply by substituting higher calorie foods such as candies with fruits and vegetables and that will make it simpler for you to attain your DASH objectives. Here are some examples:

1) - To improve Fruits: Eat a moderate apple in place of four shortbread cookies. You will save 80 calories. Eat 1/4 cup of dried apricots as opposed to a 2-ounce bag of pork rinds. It is going to save your self 230 calories.

2- To improve Veggies: consume a hamburger that has 3 oz of beef in the place of 6 oz. Insert a 1/2-cup serving of a 1/2-cup serving of egg whites. You'll save 200 calories. As an alternative of 5 oz of poultry, have a stir-fry with two oz of poultry plus 11/2 cups of fruits. Work with a little bit of vegetable oil. You'll save 50 calories.

3- To improve Fat free or low-fat dairy products: Take a 1/2-cup serving of low carb yogurt as a substitute for a 1/2-cup serving of full-fat ice-cream. You will save approximately 70 calories.

4- Additional Calorie-saving hints:

- Utilize skillet Or low-fat condiments. Use half the maximum amount of vegetable oil, either liquid or soft margarine, mayonnaise, or salad dressing table, or select available low-carb or skillet variants. Eat smaller pieces and scale gradually. Choose low-fat or low-fat dairy and dairy food. Check out the food labels to compare fat content from packed foods and items pronounced fat or low fat aren't necessarily lower in calories than their regular variants. Limit foods with a lot of additional sugar, like pies, flavored yogurts, candy bars, ice cream, sherbet, regular carbonated drinks, and fresh fruit drinks.

- Eat veggies Canned in their own juice in water. Insert fresh fruit into plain low-carb or skillet yogurt. Snack on fresh fruit, vegetable sticks, unbuttered and unsalted popcorn, or corn cakes. Drink warm water or club soda plus mix this up with a drizzle of lime or lemon.

Foods That Lower Blood-pressure

Foods that reduce Blood pressure are right at our food shop. We simply have to be aware of what they are and also to make the alternative to eat them. Therefore, just how do we understand that which foods to select? The DASH diet also has come into your rescue. The fantastic news for every one people is this eating plan isn't tricky to follow along with It lets several kinds of foods, and a lot of these, and doesn't want special or hard-to-prepare dishes.

Predicated upon your own Mediterranean Diet Plan and study by the National Heart, Lung, and Blood Institute (NHLBI), the DASH diet plan was developed by the National Institutes of Health (NIH). DASH, that stands for Dietary Approaches to Stop

Hypertension, could be your very well-researched diet to get foods that lower blood pressure that individuals have available now.

It targets on getting healthy quantities of whole grains, fish, poultry, and nuts to our daily dietplan. It permits lowfat legumes and lean red meats. Sweets and sugar-containing beverages are restricted however not expunged. This nutritious diet program is full of magnesium, potassium, and calcium and high in vegetables and fruits. Additionally, it contains higher levels of protein and fiber (18 percent). Equally vital, it requests us to put the salt shaker in order to detect yummy, healthiest strategies to season our foods.

Why We Want the DASH Diet

In accordance with research printed in a 2009 dilemma of Harvard Health Publications, around 73 million Americans and 1 billion people worldwide struggle hyper tension (the clinical term for hypertension). The NHLBI, that conducted the analysis, found a direct relationship between hypertension and cardiovascular disease, strokes, diabetes, and kidney disorder. If you are between the ages of 40 and 70, for each 20 millimeter Hg increase on your own reading or 10 millimeter Hg on your diastolic reading, then your probability of cardiovascular disease doubles.

We all know It Of those risk factors for elevated blood pressure will be eating a poor diet. Using 1 in 3 Americans coping with hypertension, the NHLBI began a report through several of their respected medical centers in the nation to find the most effective diet program for preventing or diminishing hypertension.

The analysis Consisted of a control dietplan, which symbolized the normal American dietplan, and also two additional food diets. The 3rd diet, that has been referred to as the DASH diet, also demonstrated most reliable. Their findings: blood pressure has been decreased by an eating plan That's low in Saturated-fat

Cholesterol

Absolute fat which highlights polyunsaturated or Low Fat dairy and dairy goods

The ingestion Program Also included plenty of vegetables and fruits. Health practitioners saw immediate reductions in blood pressure prices, in just a couple of weeks, in people after DASH eating plan.

The significance Of those findings can't be overestimated: Together With the DASH findings we know just how to decrease the danger of the 2 leading diet-related reasons for strokes and cardiovascular problems: cholesterol and higher blood pressure.

Another research Added a decrease in sodium (sodium) intake into the DASH program. Participants who followed the DASH program and ate 1500 milligrams (2/3 teaspoon) or less of salt each day saw a substantial further drop in their elevated blood pressure degrees.

Recommendations To get Eating Foods That Lower Blood Pressure

Eat fresh (veggies, fruits).

Create complex carbs (whole grains, such as pasta) essential to a meal.

Produce meat aside dish, not the main dish.

Eat lean meats, poultry, fish, and fish.

Eat various colours, textures, and tastes, and that means that you never become bored and return to old customs. .

Toaster, grill, roast, and stirfry; do not brush.

Eat fresh fruit and other yummy dining table sugar replacements.

Produce your mixture of seasonings to draw the tastes of food and reduce salt.

Rinse salt off in canned foods and foods that are cured if you take in them.

Alter your favorite snacks to incorporate DASH diet basics.

Make slow changes.

The DASH Diet Can Help In The Fight Against Obesity

Just like it or not The very first line of strike in fighting obesity is your conventional diet and workout program and many doctors won't consider such matters as gastric by pass operation until they're satisfied you've tried dieting and dieting badly and without the success. Thus, confronted with being forced to trek the diet down course it is sensible to decide on a diet which stands a chance of exercising out.

The DASH diet, also Which was basically developed to help lower blood pressure also can be supported by The National Heart, Lung, and Blood Institute and the The American Heart Association, is just one potential option.

Most diets concentrate Their focus on foods that you ought to avoid, requiring one to cut carbohydrates or fats such as example. Others center on the socalled dieting properties of foods that are specific and also ask that you eat copious amounts of such things . Without starting the intricacies of such food diets, the actual problem with not quite most these diets is they have been proven again and again to become inefficient. Essentially - they don't really get the job done.

What exactly makes the DASH diet plan different?

The DASH diet Focuses its attention about exactly what you should really be eating, as opposed to about which you should perhaps not be eating, also in its simplest urges eating a balance of vegetables and fruit supplemented using some low-carb milk product.

Vegetables and fruits Are great diet programs (if you eat a variety of don't only limit your self to only a couple of your favorite vegetables and fruits) for 2 chief reasons.

Fruit and Veggies contain a higher water content and are high in carbs. Which usually means you don't want to eat massive amounts of either to really feel filled and also relatively huge amounts won't supply a high calories.

Secondly, Fresh Fruit And veggies provide not just your mandatory daily intake of fiber, but can also be full of important minerals and vitamins that are crucial to keeping you healthy as you're dieting.

Whether or maybe You abide by the particular DASH diet plan or not it is quite definitely your own choice butif you're facing being forced to try out the diet and physical exercise solution for obesity, afterward an eating plan that follows the principles set out within the DASH diet plan and that concentrates its focus primarily on vegetables and fruit may be an superb path to choose.

Chapter 5: Dash Diet Food Groups

The DASH diet plan is Simple to trace because it uses common meals which are accessible at the community food shop. The DASH diet implies daily portions for each one of the various food groups. The amount of portions you take in will be dependent in your everyday caloric requirements.
Take a Look at the DASH diet here:
DASH diet Pyramid *take note: that the daily portions indicated on the basis will fluctuate based upon your caloric requirements. It is possible to locate the essential portions daily calories at the second chapter on portion control and serving sizes.
* Measure 1 - Water The maximum priority in every dietary plan is making certain you obtain the proper nutrients. A significant aspect of having the ideal nourishment comprises drinking fluids. There are several people experiencing dehydration on an everyday basis since they just don't drink enough water to maintain their organs saturated in fluids that are healthy.
The perils of dehydration
The typical Adult human body is constituted of 50 to 65 per cent water. Fat tissue doesn't contain too much water because lean tissue so that the more fat you have you personally the tougher it's for the human system to store the compulsory water required to help your organs function correctly. With your human body being contained of much water you'd believe it couldn't want anymore however that isn't correct. If one section of the human body starts to receive dry that it reduces the full flow of fluids within the human body. This reduces blood pressure by decreasing the quantity of circulation also it reduces down the blood pressure against the artery walls. While this occurs, a decrease in the quantity of oxygen from the bloodstream does occur hence lowering the oxygen levels which are attaining the critical organs and body tissues. Since it lasts,

your entire system finally begins to acquire unbalanced since it doesn't have sufficient water to maintain the fluids flowing precisely within the human physique.

Just how much water Do you really want?

In case You're Exercising and perspiration you want to improve your fluid intake to account fully for the additional loss in fluids. You ought to drink between 4 8 oz of plain water in a work out every fifteen minutes along with a second 16 ounce once you finish exercising simply to pay for the increased loss in fluids during exercising. Our bodies desire 6 4 fluid oz of water per single day to help keep them working efficiently. When your nurse has had trouble drawing blood in the human own body then decide to try drinking 6 4 fluid oz of water each and every single day per week prior to your bloodwork to determine whether it really is simpler for your blood to be attracted. 6 4 fluid ounce is equivalent to 2 - eight oz glasses of water every day.

The Way to Have The needed quantity of fluids

You Can Acquire Fluids through additional liquids besides water though maybe not all of fluids are made equal and some may harm the system should you drink a lot of these. Carbonated beverages or pops are a few samples of fluids which could harm your system. Milk, however is an adequate supply of fluid which may help you stay hydrated. It comes from next to water. It's also likely to find a number of your own water intake from vegetables, fruits and the food items that you eat. Water-Melon such as is 90 per cent water and also helps the system stay hydrated. The crux of the DASH diet is still water. A fantastic method to produce your H2O in take more appealing would be to incorporate lemon into a water together side a drop or two of liquid Stevia.

Indications of dehydration

If You like an Eight hour interval of time without draining your bladder, you're dehydrated. Symptoms of dehydration include dark urine, feeling tired, tired, moody and undergoing headaches. Whenever you're dehydrated your heart additionally must work harder to push blood through your veins. The own body will react negatively as it's to pay for a deficiency of fluids therefore make certain you remain hydrated.

Assessing your Fluid ingestion in every daily life

If you are like Me personally, you could forget to drink water during your afternoon. Fortunately there are a few fantastic alarms and software on the web which are able to remind you. Do not let something such as needing to drink a glass of plain water throughout your busy day induce one to the following aggravation. Get loads of fluids and also your own body will benefit you....plus you'll probably be reducing the strain degree in your own heart.

Tier two - Fortified Cereal, Bread, Rice, Pasta

The 2nd grade Of the DASH Diet food-pyramid comprises fortified breads, cereals, pasta and rice. Whole-grain kinds with the food collection will be most useful simply because they offer you the nourishment and contain high quantities of minerals and vitamins. Additionally they will comprise the smallest number of processed compounds including added dyes and sugars. However, what exactly do these foods do to you and how are they really going to assist you on your weight loss attempts?

Grainy meals provide energy

The grainy food Group affirms the human own body's vitality as you workforce throughout exercise or whenever you use the mind to find out something, make sure it a mathematical matter or perhaps a personal issue.

Grainy meals Keep you feeling full more

Only half a cup Of grain rice contained with a stirfry can help keep you feeling full longer than if you did not incorporate a serving of grains together with your own dinner. Eating oats for breakfast can be just a fantastic idea as they're a fantastic source of fiber. Dietary fiber leaves your intestines softer and equipped to go your pathogens together better. Breads contain fiber fiber and also behave as a naturopathic agent which will help maintain your system everyday.

Tier 3 - Veggies and Vegetables

The following class About the Dash Diet Pyramid comprises both fruits and veggies and vegetables. The starchier that the vegetable that the faster it gets you feel full and the more your sense of fullness continues. The disadvantage to starchy veggies is they develop into glucose when processed and frequently consume less water content than different kinds of veggies. Make certain that you track the dosage sizes and also perhaps not make the mistake of eating a lot of portions of starchy veggies. On the opposing hand of the DASH diet is your fresh fruit section. Rich, sweet and flavorful fruits may provide extra water into a daily diet. Additionally they fill out a pure craving most of us need for sweetness.

Vegetables and fruits Veggies are a terrific source of phyto nutrients and phyto-chemicals

Vegetables and fruits Veggies are an excellent supply of minerals and vitamins that provide the human body with the nourishment it has to combat ailments and rejuvenate your own system. The human body's source of phyto nutrients and phyto-chemicals stems out of the particular food group. Phyto-nutrients and phyto chemicals are power nutritional elements which protect you in hypertension in addition to other ailments like stroke, diabetes, cardiovascular problems and some cancers. Vegetables and fruits also allow you to keep a healthful weight since they lower cholesterol and blood pressure levels.

Eat vibrant Fruits and veggies

Eat veggies and Vegetables within a range of colors. Think "rainbow" An acronym which will be able to enable you to remember the colors of the rainbow is ROY G BIV. This Means Red, Orange, Yellow, Green, Blue, Indigo and Violet -- all of the colours of the rainbow! The more slender and much more version the colors, the more nourishment you can receive from the vegetables and fruits.

Eating more than The recommended parts

If You Decide to Eat greater than a recommended dose afterward it is ideal to eat vegetables then migrate into veggies, bear in mind that a number of veggies will become sugar in the system after you consume them. Whenever you're deficient in a certain vitamin or vitamin there's a fruit or vegetable available which comprises precisely the specific nutrient which you have to have so as to improve this lack. Adding a fruit or vegetable which you will well not eat will permit one to cover all of your nutrient foundations so you can fix your lack naturally instead of having a nutritional supplement.

Discover How to cook Your veggies and fruits

Learning the way to Cook your veggies and veggies to be able to acquire the nourishment out of their website is equally vital. The increasing loss of nourishment throughout the cooking procedure may differ with vegetables and fruits. By way of instance, cooking berries differs than just cooking different veggies since the berries nutrient worth increase the longer they're cooked. Other veggies shed most of these nutrient value once they're cooked for extended spans. Burning or ingesting veggies on high temperature causes them to drop a great deal of these nutrient value. On the flip side, allowing a garlic clove or onion to break a couple minutes once this has been sliced can boost its nutritional value. It's very good to do a little research about the best way best to cook fruits and veggies to be able to acquire the maximum nourishment out of the foods which you prepare.

Tier 4a - berry, Yogurt, Cheese

The following degree of That the DASH diet includes milk, cheese, cheese and yogurt. It stocks the particular level with meat, poultry, fish, poultry, dried beans and nuts.

The Advantages of Coffee

Dairy Solutions Are valuable since they

Help construct Longer bones and teeth

Assist the Nervous system in receiving and sending messages

Help muscles Squeeze and curl up

Help in Discharging hormones and other compounds in your system

Help preserve a Normal heartbeat

1 significant Vitamin that's associated with every one these physiological functions is calcium. Calcium is an integral ingredient in the majority of milk food.

Tier 4b - Fish, Poultry, Dry Beans and Nuts

The following degree of That the DASH diet is your meat, poultry, fish, poultry, dried beans, eggs and nuts group. This food group provides your body with iron, protein, zinc plus a vitamin-B also it keeps your system healthy and sturdy. Consistently choose lean cuts of beef and remove skin from meats such as turkey and chicken.

Advantages of the Food collection

Eggs really are an excellent Origin of protein and iron in order that is the reason why they're recorded with meats. The majority of the fat in a egg stems from the yolk thus take this under account when deciding just how many eggs to consume in one sitting. Beans are a non --fat source of nourishment. Additionally they have a high degree of fiber. Nuts are a terrific source of protein and iron plus in addition, they contain elevated quantities of very good fat.

Tier 5 - Fats, Oils, Sweets, Supplements

The Maximum grade To the food market could be your oils, fats, sweets and supplements set. Each thing within this food collection is always to be used . Opposite that's the magnesium, vitamin D, vitamin D, vitamin b 12 and nutritional supplement set. The DASH diet suggests adding calcium, calcium, vitamin D and vitamin b 12 to your everyday regimen because the majority of individuals are with a lack of those vitamins and also the increasing loss in these minerals because we all age suggests the significance of an extra nutritional supplement for all these particular nutritional elements.

Select Your oils And fats sensibly

When picking Minerals and fats that you want to choose sensibly. Omega3 and omega6 essential fatty acids are called "essential" fatty acids as your human body can't produce them by itself. You may just get them . These fats reduce inflammation and protect against cardiovascular disease. You get those fats mostly from nuts, fish and certain forms of veggies. Fully processed foods have a great deal of oils and fats as well but these aren't the most useful types of oils and fats to eat up.

Just how much fat, how Carbohydrates, cholesterol and protein does this DASH diet plan allow? Overall fat - 27 percent
Polyunsaturated fats - 6 percent
Carbs - 55 percent of your calories daily
Protein - 18 percent Of your calories
Cholesterol - 150-mg

Chapter 6: Portion Control And Serving Sizes

The DASH dietary emphasizes the significance of portion size, eating an assortment of foods and securing the ideal quantity of nourishment. Frequently it isn't exactly what you eat that's that the issue rather it's just how much you consume. Yes...measuring the meal so you eat balanced portions through the entire afternoon of each and every food group is sometimes described as a job but it's critical. Therefore how can you build the practice of measuring parts out each time you eat? I began wearing store purchased packs quite a very long time past and found I actually re-packaged foods at horribly massive amounts for my families demanded serving sizes. Like I re-packaged food I'd tell myself I had to make certain I cooked and I had enough for left overs. Then I began watching that which we did with all the additional portions which I had repackaged. Ordinarily, we did not utilize them for that which I'd planned and ate significantly more than we have to have. It's astonishing to learn what you need verses everything you truly **eat are** just two different matters. My spouse's investigation as a parasitic gradually transferred us right into a brand new age of eating from our loved ones. His heart attack and insulin problems that converted to our daily diet challenges became our principal cause of learning new behaviors.

Learning how to see packs earlier I purchased foods became extremely essential. Are the food worth eating? In what looked like each day that my worth worth suddenly shifted. My eyes started to open into the need for choosing high nutritional supplements as opposed to foods which offered little to no nutrition. I began measuring snacks out in to portion sizes and repackaging them to zip loc bags. This worked well as you did not need to complete the math once you wanted a bite. It had been figured out. I broke our beef bundles right into two three and four separate meal plans as opposed to earning extra in a couple of meals. I came across that bites were meals and snacks were meals. There is a period when my husband could earn a dual --decker sandwich to get a bite! Those days are behind us today and we all realize a bite is merely that, a bite. The most useful information I could provide would be to begin your own "portion size re-packaging efforts" with the meals that you now have from the pantry, freezer and refrigerator. Whenever you get started reviewing serving sizes you can find a number of things which will certainly surprise you concerning just what a serving size happens to be.

Learn on your Foods and also the procedures taken to receive them to promote. You might discover that buying fruit and cutting on yourself permits one to eat more fresh fruit. Why? Because processing comprises additives which drive the calories up while still reducing dosage dimensions. When veggies are canned they often times require sugar for a preservative. This aids the percentage size. Additionally, whenever you buy oats using real fresh fruit that the yogurt may comprise extra additives which the maker had to increase the yogurt to maintain the fresh fruit from spoiling. That is generally a sugar-based syrup of some type. It's really a better option to purchase plain yogurt and insert your own fresh fruit into it.

DASH diet Allowable calories and portions

The DASH diet Plan indicates the subsequent portions each day of each food category. There are 3 distinct metabolic degrees therefore portions are corrected to accommodate each degree.

1600 Calories a Day:

Grains (rather whole grains or Multi-grains) = 6 servings

Veggies = 3 - 4 portions

Fruits = 4 servings

Fat--liberated or Low-fat milk and dairy goods = 2 - 3 portions

Liver Organ, Fish and poultry 3 - 4 (or fewer) portions

Seeds, seeds, Beans = three or four portions each week
Fats and oils respectively. 2 servings
Sweets and additional Sugars = 3 or more servings each week
2600 Calories a Day:
Grains (rather whole grains or Multi-grains) = 10 - 1 1 portions
Veggies = 5 - 6 servings
Berries = 5 - 6 servings
Fat free or Low-fat milk and dairy goods = 3 portions

Liver Organ, Fish and poultry 6 servings
Seeds, seeds, Beans = 1. serving
Fats and oils respectively. 3 portions
Sweets and additional Sugars as many as 2 portions each day however, not mandatory
3100 Calories a Day:
Grains (rather whole grains or Multi-grains) = 1-2 - 1-3 portions
Veggies = 6 servings
Fruits = 6 servings
Fatfree or Low-fat milk and dairy goods = three or four portions
Liver Organ, Fish and poultry 6 - 9 portions
Seeds, seeds, Beans = 1. serving
Fats and oils respectively. 4 portions
Sweets and additional Sugars as many as 2 portions each day however, not mandatory

Dash Diet Food List

Veggies Low-Glycemic Veggies (Make them your initial option)
Avocados, Arugula, Artichokes, Asparagus, Brussels sprouts Broccoli, Bell peppers, Celery Cabbage, Cauliflower, Cucumbers, Collard greens, Eggplant, Green beans, Kale, Lettuce (the darker that the leafy green, the greater) Mustard greens, and Mushrooms, Onions, Radishes, Spinach, Snow peas, Swiss chard, Summer squash, Sprouts, Turnip greens, and Zucchini
Higher Glycemic Veggies (Make them your next option) Acorn skillet

Butternut squash Chickpeas, Carrots, English legumes, citrus lettuce, Spaghetti squash Tomatoes

Not permitted: White berries Corn

Fruits

Lower-glycemic Fruits (First option) All fruits are all permitted; Apricots, Apples, Blackberries, Blueberries, Bananas, Cranberries, Casaba melon, Cantaloupe, Grapes, Guavas, Honeydew melon, Limes, Lemons, Nectarines, Peaches, Papayas, Rhubarb, Raspberries, Strawberries, Watermelons

Higher Glycemic Fruits (Second-choice)
Cherries, Figs, Grapefruits, Kiwis, Mango, Oranges, Plums, Pears, Pumpkin, Tangerines

Meats and Seafood

All shellfish, All fish (particularly fatty fish such as salmon, mackerel sardines and so on), Steak, (select lean roasts and legumes and additional lean ground beef), Chicken (skinless), Eggs, Game birds and legumes, Lamb (lean), Pork (lean roasts and legumes), Turkey (skinless and floor), Turkey bacon (low sodium)

Not permitted: Bacon (routine), Cold cuts packed and deli meats, Jerky, Sausage

Dairy

Almond-milk, Blue cheese, Cheddar and Cottage-cheese (Lowfat), Cow's milk (1 percent and skim), Cream-cheese (Lowfat), Feta-cheese, Greek yogurt, Margarine or butter substitute, Parmesan cheese (High-sodium in order restrict), Mozzarella cheese, Provolone cheese (low carb), Routine yogurt (low carb), Ricotta cheese (Lowfat), Soy-milk, Sour-cream (low carb), Swiss-cheese

Not permitted: Full-fat legumes, curry, cheese,

Fats

Almonds, Black Walnuts, Brazil nuts, Canola oil, flax seed oil, jojoba or Margarine substitute, Mayonnaise (low carb), Pecans, Olives (low-sodium), coconut oil, Sesame seeds, sun flower seeds

Not permitted: Olive oil, sesame oil, along with the Other vegetable oils

Grains

Almond flour Brown-rice Barley Coconut flour Wheat-germ Whole Grain bread Wholegrain low-carb cold cereal Wholegrain blended grain hot cereal Wholegrain pita Whole Grain lean bagel Whole Grain steel-cut oats Whole Grain lean British noodles Whole Wheat flour Wholegrain tortillas

Not permitted: Corn muffins Corn bread Cornmeal Oatmeal (instant or roasted) Sweetened cold peppers

Condiments, Seasonings and "additional"

Almond butter Agave nectar Coffee Caesar dressing, Dressing (low sodium or some sodium) Flax Seed Flaxseed oil Herbs Spices Hot sauce Honey-mustard (not Honey-mustard) Preserves (low or no glucose) Peanut-butter (limitation) Jellies (low or no sugar) Quinoa Sesame butter Salsa Pickles (sour and dill) Soy sauce (low sodium) Teriyaki sauce (low sodium) Tea (cold or hot) Tomato of skillet (no sugar) Chicken, vegetable or beef broth (no or low sodium) Vinaigrette Whey protein powder (no sugar added) Soy protein powder

Not permitted: Alfredo sauce (ready) Cheese sauce (ready) Gravies (ready) Mayonnaise (total --fat) Barbeque, beef and other leftovers (low to normal sodium)

Sweet Treats

Dried fruits (no more Sugar included) Fudge pops (fatfree) Frozen fruit bars (no sugar added) Gelatin Ice cream (low carb) 1. oz square-foot chocolate Pudding (fat free) Popsicles Sorbet Sherbet

Chapter 7: Employing Dash To Shed Weight

Unlike programs in Other books which line book store shelves, the app isn't planning to coach you on just how exactly to "diet" Failed concepts like nutrient dividing or accelerated weight loss don't have any invest DASH. Long-term fat loss requires lifestyle changes instead of gimmick dieting. The fact is, DASH boosts a wholesome life style, and fat loss is really a really wonderful complication! DASH is targeted on food, for example fresh fruits and veggies, elaborate whole grains, healthful milk, and lean meats at proper percentage to advertise gratification and increased energy through the time, minus the possibility of over eating. There's therefore much to profit by learning to be a DASHer: fat loss, energy advantage, and increased immunity to chronic diseases top the list.

DASH Can Make it Simple to shed excess weight and keep it off by teaching how to choose sensibly. It isn't an issue of only adhering to an idea, even though that'll undoubtedly help in the start, but of knowing how to get healthful decisions. Education, together with the resources and tools to take actions, permits realistic execution of changes and also clears the road to goal conclusion. The recipes in this publication are intended to create cooking healthful meals yummy and simple, without sacrificing favorite foods and tastes. Incorporating exercise into a regular routine will donate to major and sustainable change. The previous section in this publication is really a 28-day DASH meal program, helping to make it simple to know that the essentials of healthful eating and cooking in order that customs actually change.

Calorie Needs For Weight loss

Before starting A healthier weight reduction program, it is crucial to get a starting point or baseline. There are numerous techniques to figure a wholesome weight. Body Mass Index (BMI) is a measure of body fat based on weight and height reduction. The formulation

For calculating BMI is:
Weight (pound) ÷ [height (in)2] × 703
Truth: Weight = 165 pounds, Height = 5' 8" (6-8")
Calculation: [165 ÷ (6-8)two] × 703 = 25.09
BMI Isn't a Specific science. Quick and cheap, it delivers an indicator of excess weight. In general, the BMI of somebody at a healthful weight should fall between 19 and 25. Waist circumference is just another quick method to test whether somebody are at a wholesome weight. Broadly speaking, waist circumference ought to be greater than 35 1.es for females, and also less than 40 1.es for males. Calculating the proportion of your body fat is really a little harder as it is not something which could be achieved in your home. Technically body fat is your whole burden of an individual's fat separated by the individual's weight, also is made up of important body storage and fat human body fat. The several procedures and tools useful to calculate body weight percent include (but aren't confined to) calipers, infra red lighting, x ray ab-sorptiometry, water displacement, bioelectrical impedance analysis, and anthropometric procedures. Wholesome body weight percentages for mature women is 15 to 22 percent, also for mature men 8 to 15 percent.
Now, to begin Making modifications: The nutrition program is predicated on 2000 calories each day, that will be meant for men and women that are emotionally active. Make use of the 1,200 calorie every day alteration if exercise isn't really a part of one's own plan. Don't eat up under 1,200 calories a day; your system requires at the least 1000 calories every day for manhood functioning independently. Some times decreasing

caloric consumption to 2,000 calories each day can be too much of a jump for folks. If that's the scenario, try to lower your daily calories simply by only 500 each day. For those who don't have any clue just how many calories you are taking in, then simply stick to the 2000 calorie every day program, addin a lot of those nutritious snacks which can be recorded, and then work your way right down to just 2000 each day.

DASH Weightless Guidelines

Gut your own refrigerator. After DASH necessitates consuming fully processed foods and crap. The perfect method to prevent consuming these things is to eradicate them! Replace the fully processed food items using genuine food: fruits, fresh veggies and fruits, raw nuts, and whole grains. When it's simply a lot of time to throw all of the terrible stuff simultaneously, then stop buying it therefore you phase it from their kitchen as time passes.

Produce a grocery List for your own supermarket and farmer's market. Before you go into the current market, have a list of DASH friendly foods to that weekly meal plans. This prep helps maintain tempting foods in bay. Realize the most of these DASH friendly foods can be found on the outside of the supermarket. Steer clear of the heart ducks, where tens of thousands of depleted fully processed food items can be found.

Cook in house Whenever potential. Even when it appears healthy, foods prepared in restaurants might be full of a great deal of extra calories without even fundamentally providing additional satisfaction or nourishment. There's no solution to restrain both the ingredients used along with even the preparation of food you never create your self. Whenever you cook in your home, you've got total control on the type and caliber of one's meal, in addition to how it's prepared and just how much you eat. It's a lot simpler to learn nutrition labels and create healthful decisions whenever you look for food and prepare it yourself.

Start Looking for DASH foods. Create a mind set that repeats DASH food items. Figure out methods to add fresh fruit in your dinner or lunch. Insert a dose of steamed vegetables into your own meal, and then spare the remaining most important path for after. In restaurants, arrange a side of vegetables rather than fries.

Choose Restaurants and cafes which have DASH foods readily available to purchase. Finally the unfriendly locations will be desired.

Stock-pile that your Kitchen and office. Continue to keep your freezer, pantry, and icebox full of DASH foods in order to prevent injuries. Maintain loads of freshly cut veggies and fruits together with nuts and legumes hand to get snacks and quick meals on the move. Stock any office refrigerator, also, therefore that there are always healthy selections out there.

Obtain a deal on Percentage control. Our society has become a"super size me" universe, in more ways than you. Most restaurants serve just two to three servings each meal, so a lot more than is needed at one single sitting. It's easy to fall prey to the exercise in your home, too. We get prepared to large pieces and eating a great deal. We utilize big bowls, plates, and glassware and then fill up them. To prevent overeating, then follow the dimensions while in the DASH meal program. Make use of an electronic digital scale to quantify and soon you know correct portion sizes.

Dash-Friendly Restaurant Guidelines

• Order a to Go Box together with your mealand put 1 / 2 the food away the moment it arrives. Once the food has gone out of sight, then you are not as inclined to over eat.

• Split up Appetizers, entrées, and desserts along with family and friends. Surprisingly, most of those"half of" portions are in reality regularized servings.

• Divide a bigger Salad.

- Ask Restaurants to provide you dressing table, dressing, toppings, and sauces on the other side. Eat a very small part of these extras, either or none in any way.
- Ask the waiter Perhaps not to attract bread in the meal. Bread-and-butter add up promptly. Save calories to the meal.
- Eat slowly. Dine with the others in order that eating pops together with dialog. You'll eat up less you decrease, and you're going to have a much better grip on whenever you are full. Drink water through your meal to fill out.
- Prevent carbonated Drinks, such as alcohol, together with meals. Carbonated beverages may very quickly package an extra 500 to 1000 calories on meals!
- Alternatively of Dessert, choose a glass of wine or coffee after a dinner. There are a lot fewer calories at those beverages than at a standard restaurant supper, yet you're still able to delight in a post-meal treat.
- Avoid fast Food restaurants fully. There's nearly always another alternative. Quick food is filled up with processed ingredients also it is prepared for volume, not quality. It's doubtful as to if it's technically food! Its empty calories contribute to weight reduction.

Exercise

Exercise Can Be an Integral part of DASH-recommended life style varies. It'll give rise to fat reduction, lower blood pressure, and reduced risk of a number of different chronic diseases like diabetes and even cancer. Making exercise part of your life style can allow you to get the outcomes that you wish to attain. Exercise contains three chief components: cardiovascular fitness, resistance training, and endurance. Each component is just as vital for burning fat and slimming down by boosting metabolic rate and increasing muscles. Cardio vascular training strengthens the center and reduces both systolic and diastolic blood pressure levels. Additionally, it increases metabolic process as time passes, meaning your body will burn off calories faster and better. Begin aerobic exercise gradually and raise the strength as you build endurance.

A Fantastic Way to Start is by simply walking thirty minutes every day. Walk , increasing your heart rate and breathing speed, to make sure a fantastic work out. (When necessary, start out with only 10 to 15 minutes and work around half an hour.) Since your endurance grows, add other cardio vascular activities like running, stair climbing, bicycling, aerobic classes, hiking, or dance. Cardio vascular exercise includes something which involves human anatomy movement and that increases heart rate and breath rate. For weight reduction, you ought to do vigorous aerobic exercise to get at least half an hour at one time, three or even four times every week. Resistance training, or weight training, helps get rid of fat quickly by increasing muscle mass and boosting metabolic rate. Resistance training is crucial so as to attain weightloss targets. Resistance training could be achieved in your home, outdoors, or even at the gymnasium.

Like Cardiovascular workout, start slowly. In the beginning, simply use your body weight for weight training together with motions such as lunges, squats, pushups, and stomach exercises. Since the own body potency increases, add intensity and weights into workout. Vary work-outs by making use of local tools for weight training classes, outdoor bootcamps, or even individual trainers. For maximum weight outcome, resistance workout sessions should continue at least half an hour four times every week. High-intensity workouts center on extending and balance. This aspect can be overlooked but is equally as crucial as strength-training exercise. Stretching helps prevent injury during and after exercise, even by simply allowing joints and muscles to heat up until workouts and recuperate then. Before working outside, warm up your muscles for approximately five full minutes by knowingly extending them. Do enormous moves, such like arm bands, leg swings, and cool bands, or jump rope.

After functioning Out, require 5 to 10 minutes to elongate the muscles that you used throughout your work out session. Such a stretching involves extending the muscles used throughout the work out simply by holding the stretch for many seconds to many minutes. Exercising also supplies invaluable time to sign in with the own body and pay attention to exactly what it's needs. Balance exercises help work miniature strengthening muscles which influence posture and equilibrium, you need to comprise performing exercises on unstable surfaces. One-legged exercises and usage of fitness balls, foam rollers, wobble boards, and also BOSU balls really are typical cases of exercises.

Exercise Reviews and Suggestions

Five occasions per Week

Cardio Vascular. Start with walking for thirty minutes. If you are pushed for a while or possess some physical limits, break this up to three 10-minute periods. Walk so that your pulse and breathing rate increase. You ought to feel like you should be training! As your endurance improves, increase and alter the strength of your workouts by simply incorporating such exercises like cycling, running, stair climbing, hiking, swimming pool, and rock-climbing. Exercise for 30 to 60 minutes for greatest effects.

Stretching. Before walking, then warm up your joints and muscles by doing arm swings after which leg swings to get an overall total of two to three minutes. After walking stretch by elongating the muscles holding the stretch for 1 or 2 minutes to every single stretch. Stretching helps prevent injury and boosts flexibility.

3 X per week Week

Strength Training. Give attention to training enormous muscles like the ones from the thighs, chest, back, as well as heart. Focus on your body weight for resistance, then add extra weight and strength as your own stamina assembles. Do high-intensity workouts daily, resting the huge muscles between workouts.

Focus training. Incorporate balance training in your resistance practice through the use of equipment like fitness center balls, wobble boards, foam rollers, and BOSU balls and from doing exercises that are aerobic.

Stretching. After equilibrium or strength training, then stretch by elongating the muscles holding the stretch for 1 or two minutes to every single stretch. It certainly is hard to start a brand new life style addiction, like working from a normal basis, particularly when you can find hundreds and hundreds of reasons to not exercise. Below are a few recommendations to keep you on target.

- Obtain an Liability partner. This individual can work out together with you personally, or simply check in with one each day to be certain that you're staying on the right track.
- Take Note of Your own targets and find how you are doing weekly.
- Maintain an Exercise diary to record your daily successes and beats also to track your own progress.
- Produce a Routine to ensure exercising becomes part of one's everyday pursuits.
- Conserve some time and Money by training in your home. You're able to cause a home gymnasium, or even follow workout routines readily available on the web, on television, or even on DVD. There are various free resources.
- workout in The afternoon, so you do not go out of time through your afternoon and also you start every daytime energized.
- Use the Of local tools such as classes, bootcamps, and individual coaches, and that means you've got an instructor advising and inspiring you.
- Employ a Personal trainer to generate ideal workouts for both you too as hold you liable for doing this.
- Produce a songs Play list that motivates one to exercise.
- Invest Workout clothing which allow you to feel well.
- Consistently have Water that you remain energized and hydrated through the duration of your work out. (steer clear from sugar-filled or sweetened energy or work out beverages)

* Caution: Should You've got hypertension or some chronic illness, ask your primary care doctor before starting a workout regime. Your physician needs to perform a physical examination of one's physical fitness level before starting any strenuous activity.

Chapter 8: Dash-Friendly Recipes

Experienced DASHers Will inform you they eat at home more frequently than not. Cooking for your self and your loved ones provides you invaluable control on what goes to your own diet, also makes it a lot easier to make healthier decisions. Whenever another person prepares your own food, you do not understand just what's inside it. That you never know more about the product quality or freshness of the ingredients, if they are organic, if they truly are processed, or whether damaging additives are found. Additionally you lose some control on size, and it is an essential facet of DASH. There are various advantages to cooking in your home for friends and family: it takes one to plan and utilize healthful ingredients, and also to participate with other individuals. Certainly it's not possible to eat each and every meal in your home, however the more food you really do eat in your home, the better you're stay glued to DASH and the improved results you'll find. Most the recipes in this publication were written and analyzed by Anna V. Zulaica, owner and chef of Presto! Catering and Food Services, situated in the San Francisco Bay Area Bay Region.

Since you browse Throughout the recipes, so bear in your mind you always need to use organic, fresh, unprocessed ingredients whenever you can. Salt is kept to the absolute minimum from the meals ("a p1.," as an instance, is significantly less than 1/8 tsp), also if it's contained, it's in the sort of seasalt, and this will be less processed than just table salt also comprises valuable minerals. Nut butters utilized from the recipes are consistently the raw selection. The feel of this nut-butter, while it's smooth or crispy, just isn't defined since it's dependent upon your own taste. Lots of recipes contain serving hints, healthy tips and recommendations, or recipe modifications. Optional ingredients are occasionally mentioned, but take be aware they are not included within the nutrition facts because of this recipe. Nutrition facts, recorded for each recipe, also comprise information regarding carbs, fats, carbs, fiber, sugar, protein, and also the minerals potassium, sodium, phosphorus, and calcium.

Smoothies

Smoothies are a Quick, simple, and flavorful solution to fit additional portions of produce to daily, plus so they're fantastic for on the go snacks and meals packaged with vitamins, fiber, minerals, antioxidants, and healthful fats. Experiment using fruit and veggie mixes to locate your favorite smoothie!

Smoothie Guidelines:

- Many recipes Call for greens. Make sure you combine them with a little liquid before adding different ingredients into an own blender, therefore that their fibrous feel rests .
- Spinach is your Many neutral-tasting green you're able to enhance your smoothie, also it's really a good one to begin with if you are reluctant about green beverages. Then experimentation using various greens to detect their tastes and tastes.
- Some recipes call for new fruit, the others fruit. Frozen and fresh fruit might be used responsibly. Just remember that frozen fresh fruit will make a frostier, thicker, more colder smoothie compared to fruit.

- When Purchasing dried fresh fruit, buy organic and steer clear of sugar. • Adding ice hockey is one other means to acquire yourself a thicker, frostier smoothie.
- Peanut or Almond butter, avocado, coconut, and coconut oil are all healthy fats you can enhance your smoothie. Not only does one feel fuller more using those ingredients, but also the wholesome fat helps the body digest and absorb minerals out of the vegetables.

- Smoothies can Be kept in the fridge for 24 hours. In case the smoothie divides into layers throughout heat, simply stir before drinking.
- Consistently comprise At the very least one serving of vegetables on your own smoothie to make sure you're getting valuable minerals together side the vitamins from fresh fruit, also to balance the sour fruit information. (Normally vegetables are high in minerals, where as fresh fruit is significantly high in vitamins.)

Blueberry Green Smoothie

- Serves 2
- 2 cups sliced blended Greens (such as kale, collard greens, mustard greens, Swiss chard, and lettuce)
- 1/4 cup water
- 1/3 cup sliced carrot
- 1/2 cup suspended blueberries
- 1/2 cup coarsely chopped unpeeled cucumber
- 1/4 cup Un-sweetened almond-milk
- 4 Ice

Set the greens And water in a blender. Start blending in low, so that whilst the greens start to break down, slowly grow to moderate speed until they have been completely divided and smooth. Bring the remaining ingredients, and mix medium to high speed until desired consistency is achieved, about 1 second. Drink instantly.

Papaya Goodness

- Serves 2
- 1 cup lettuce 1 Cup chopped spinach
- 3/4 cup water
- 1/2 cup sliced unpeeled cucumber
- 1 apple cider, coarsely chopped
- 1 cup coarsely Chopped pineapple
- 1 tbsp Ground flax seed

Set the spinach, Lettuce water in a blender. Start blending in low, so that whilst the greens start to break up, grow to moderate speed until they have been completely divided and smooth. Bring the remaining ingredients, and mix medium to high speed until desired consistency is achieved, about 1 second. Drink instantly.

Wakeup call!

- Serves 2
- 1 big rib celery,
- Chopped 1. Tbsp fresh parsley
- 1/2--3/4 cup Water
- 1/2 cup sliced Cooked beets
- 1 orange, Split into sections
- 3/4 cup sliced carrot

Place the Celery, carrot, and warm water in a blender. Start blending in low, so that the carrot and carrot start to break up, increase to moderate speed until they have been completely divided and smooth. Bring the remaining ingredients, and mix medium to high speed until desired consistency is achieved, about 1 second. Drink instantly.

Diabetic-Friendly Green Smoothie

- Serves 2
- 2 cups spinach
- 2 big kale leaves,
- Chopped (approximately 1 1/2 cups)
- 3/4 cup water Large skillet,
- Chopped 1/2 cup Frozen blossom
- 1/2 cup suspended peach
- 1 tbsp Ground flax seeds
- 1 tbsp Almond butter or peanut butter, discretionary

Place the Spinach, spinach, and warm water in a blender. Start blending in low, so that whilst the greens start to break up, grow to moderate speed until they have been broken down and slick. Insert the fresh fruit, flax seeds, and then nut butter (if using), and then mix medium to high speed until desired consistency is reached, about 1 second. Drink instantly.

Banana Almond Smoothie

- Serves 1.
- 1 large banana
- 1 cup Un-sweetened almond-milk
- 1 tbsp Unsalted vanilla butter
- 1 tbsp Wheat germ

- 1/8 tsp vanilla extract
- 1/8 tsp ground cinnamon
- 3--4 Ice cubes

Place all of the ingredients in a blender. Start blending in low, and also whilst the contents start to break up, grow to moderate speed until desired consistency is reached, about 1 second. Drink instantly.

Tropical Smoothie

- Serves Two
- 3/4 cup suspended mango
- 3/4 cup suspended Pine-apple
- 1 little rooted Banana, sliced
- 1 1/2 cups unsweetened coconut milk
- 1/2 cup water
- 1 tbsp Coconut oil
- 3--4 Ice cubes

Place all of the ingredients in a blender. Start blending in low, so that whilst the contents start to break up, increase to moderate speed until completely smooth, approximately 1 minute. Drink instantly.

Berry Banana Green Smoothie

- Serves Two

- 2 cups spinach
- 1 cup water
- 3/4 cup suspended blackberries
- 3/4 cup suspended blueberries
- 1 little rooted Banana, sliced
- 1 tbsp Vanilla butter

Place the Water and lettuce in a blender. Start blending in low, so that the spinach begins to break up, increase to moderate speed until it's completely broken down and smooth. Insert the blackberries, blueberries, banana, and vanilla butter and mix medium to high speed until desired consistency is achieved, about 1 second. Drink instantly.

Peach Green Smoothie

- Serves Two
- 2 cups spinach
- 1 cup water
- 1/2 cup suspended Berries
- 1 1/2 cups Frozen cherry
- 1 little rooted Banana, sliced
- 1 tbsp Coconut oil

Place the Water and lettuce in a blender. Start blending in low, so that the spinach begins to divide, grow to moderate rate until it's completely broken down and smooth. Insert the coconut and fruit oil, and then mix medium to high speed until desired consistency is achieved, about 1 second. Drink instantly.

Green Avocado Smoothie

- Serves Two
- 1 cup sliced kale
- 3/4--1 cup water.
- 1 apple cider, Chopped
- 2 little kiwifruit, peeled and halved
- 1 small avocado, Pitted, peeled, and sliced
- 1 tangerine, Peeled and divided into sections
- 3--4 Icecubes

Put the kale And water in a blender. Start blending in low, so that since the spinach begins to break down, slowly grow to moderate speed until it's completely divided and smooth. Bring the remaining ingredients, and mix medium to high speed until desired consistency is achieved, about 1 second. Drink instantly.

Melon Mélange

- Serves Two
- 2 cups spinach
- 1/2--3/4 cup Water
- 1/2 cup suspended Berries
- 3/4 cup sliced Honey dew melon
- 3/4 cup sliced cantaloupe
- 1 tbsp Ground flax seeds
- 3--4 Icecubes

Place the Water and lettuce in a blender. Start blending in low, so that the spinach begins to break up, increase to moderate speed until it's completely broken down and smooth. Insert the fresh fruit, flax seeds, and ice cream, and blend on medium to high speed until desired consistency is reached, about 1 second. Drink instantly.

Strawberry Cucumber De Light

- Serves Two
- 1 1/2 cups Frozen berries
- 2 cups sliced unpeeled cucumber
- Juice of 1/2 Large orange
- 4 mint leaves
- 3/4 cup water
- 3--4 Icecubes

Place all of the ingredients in a blender. Start blending in low, so that whilst the contents start to break up, increase to moderate speed until desired consistency is reached, about 1 second. Drink instantly.

Pump-Kin Pie Smoothie

- Serves Two
- 1/2 cup pumpkin puree
- 1/2 big rooted Banana, sliced
- 1/2 cup water
- 1 cup Un-sweetened almond-milk
- 1/4 tsp ground cinnamon
- 1/8 tsp soil nutmeg
- 1 tbsp pure maple syrup
- 3--4 Icecubes

Place the Pumpkin, banana, and warm water in a blender. Start blending in low, so that whilst the ingredients start to break up, increase to moderate speed until completely divided and smooth. Bring the remaining ingredients, and mix medium to high speed until desired consistency is achieved, about 1 second. Drink immediately.

Arugula Smoothie

- Serves Two
- 1 cup arugula
- 1 cup lettuce
- --1 1/2 cups Water
- 1/2 little banana
- 1 cup sliced Berries
- 1/2 cup blueberries
- 1 tbsp Coconut oil
- 1 tbsp Wheat germ
- 3--4 Ice cubes

Place the Arugula, spinach, and warm water in a blender. Start blending in low, and also whilst the greens start to break up, grow to moderate rate until they have been completely divided and smooth. Insert the fresh fruit, coconut oil, wheatgerm, and ice cream, and blend on medium to high speed until desired consistency is achieved, about 1 second. Drink instantly.

Chapter 9: Dash Break-Fast

It is accurate: Breakfast may be the main meal of their afternoon. Eating meals at the daytime jumpstarts your metabolic rate to the afternoon, and with no, your metabolic rate will stay lethargic and down. (Your Metabolic Rate decides the speed at which you burn off Calories) Eating dinner in an hour of stirring helps to ensure your system gets the fuel it has get started and take you during your afternoon. These healthy, fresh, quick recipes really are an excellent solution to begin daily, and give an alternate to smoothies.

Stinks Using Almond Butter And Banana

- Serves 1
- 2 pieces 100 percent Whole wheat bread
- 2 tbsp Vanilla butter
- 1 small banana, also sliced
- 1/8 tsp ground cinnamon
- Toast bread, And spread each piece with vanilla butter. Arrange the banana slices at the top, and then sprinkle with cinnamon.

English Muffin Using Berries

- Serves 1
- 100% complete Wheat English muffin, halved
- 1 tbsp Lowfat cream-cheese
- 4 berries, Thinly sliced

- 1/2 cup blueberries, mashed
- Toast the English muffin halves. Spread the cream evenly onto each toasted half and top with the fresh fruit.
- Healthy "Lox" English Muffin
- Serves Two
- 100% complete Wheat English muffin, halved
- 1/4 tsp Finely chopped fresh dill
- 1/2 tsp Fresh lemon juice
- 2 tbsp Lowfat cream-cheese
- (4-ounce) may Wild salmon in plain water, no salt added, drained
- 6 thin pieces unpeeled cucumber
- 6 thin pieces Roma tomato
- Oily black pepper

Toast the English muffin halves. In a smaller bowl mix the chopped dill and lemon juice evenly in the cream . Spread the cream cheese mixture evenly on every single muffin half. Rinse the salmon under flowing water to eliminate the liquid that is canned, then scoop the salmon equally on the English muffin halves. When the salmon is still overly big, mash with fork . Top with tomato and cucumber pieces, and sprinkle with pepper to taste.

Protein Bowl

- Serves 1.
- 3/4 cup Low Fat Cottage cheese
- 1/2 moderate Ginger, thinly chopped

- 1 tbsp Vanilla butter
- 1/4 cup raw Historical oats

Mix each of the Ingredients together in a little bowl, and also enjoy instantly.

Berries De Luxe Oatmeal

- Serves Two
- 1 1/2 cups Unsweetened almond milk
- 1/8 tsp vanilla extract
- 1 cup Historical oats
- 3/4 cup blend of blueberries, blackberries, and coarsely chopped
- Berries
- 2 tbsp toasted pecans

Heating the almond Vanilla and milk in a small sauce pan on medium heat. Once the mix begins to Simmer, add the ginger and simmer for approximately four minutes, or until the majority of the liquid Is consumed. Stir in the berries. Scoop the mixture to 2 bowls, and best with toasted pecans.

Apples And Cinnamon Oatmeal

- Serves Two
- 1 1/2 cups Unsweetened almond milk
- 1 cup Historical oats
- 1 large unpeeled Granny Smith apple, cubed
- 1/4 tsp ground cinnamon
- 2 tbsp Toasted walnut bits

Bring the milk To a simmer over moderate heat, and then add the apple and ginger cider. Stir until the majority of the liquid is absorbed, approximately 4 minutes. Stir in the cinnamon. Scoop the oatmeal mix to two bowls, and top with walnuts.

Energy Oatmeal

- Serves 1.
- 1/4 cup water
- 1/4 cup Low Fat milk
- 1/2 cup Historical oats
- 4 egg whites, beaten
- 1/8 tsp ground cinnamon
- 1/8 tsp Ground ginger
- 1/4 cup blueberries

In a small bud, Heat the milk and water to a simmer on medium heat. Insert the oats, stirring for approximately four seconds, or until the majority of the liquid is consumed. Add the crushed egg whites gently, stirring frequently. Cook for another five minutes, or until the eggs are not runny. Pour the cinnamon and ginger in to the oatmeal mix, and then simmer the mixture to a bowl. Top of tomatoes and serve immediately.

Anna's Homemade Granola

- Serves 1 2 (Makes 5-- 5 6 cups)
- 3 cups Historical oats
- 1/4 cup Flax seeds
- 1 cup sliced almonds

- 1/2 tsp ground cinnamon
- 1/4 tsp Ground ginger
- 1/4 cup brownish Sugar
- 1/4 cup walnut Honey or syrup
- 1/4 cup additional Jojoba oil
- 1/2 tsp Vanilla infusion
- 1 cup gold raisins
- Olive oil spray

Preheat the oven Into 250°F. In a big bowl combine the first six ingredients and mix to incorporate well. In a different small bowl mix together the maple syrup or oil, honey, and vanilla extract. Pour the wet ingredients to the dry components and
Mix evenly together with A spatula until you can find really no further arid stains. Pour two greased jar. Bake for approximately 1 hour and fifteen minutes, stirring every 15 minutes to realize an additional color. Since you stir fry, divide chunks of granola into the specified consistency. Remove from the oven and move to a bowl. Stir in the sausage in order that they disperse evenly.
TIPS
• Should You Would like Raisins dryer and chewier, put them into the mix before baking.
• Substitute Dried berries, cherries, or apricots for sandwiches for an assortment of tastes, colors, and anti oxidants.
• Substitute Vanilla extract for vanilla extract, even if you prefer.

• Maple-syrup And honey possess different flavor profiles however may be used properly in this recipe.
• Store chilled Granola in large zip-top cupboards or glass containers .

Warm Quinoa Using Berries

- Serves Two
- 1 cup raw quinoa
- 1 cup unsweetened coconut milk
- 1 cup water
- 1/2 cup blackberries
- 2 tbsp toasted chopped pecans
- 2 tsp raw Honey, discretionary

Rinse the quinoa (if maybe not prerinsed). At a little covered pot, bring the quinoa, almond water and milk to a boil over high temperature. Reduce heat to low and simmer for 10 to 15 minutes or until the liquid was consumed. Cooked quinoa ought to be marginally al dente; it really is ready when the majority of the grains have uncoiled and you're able to start to see the unwound germ. Enable the quinoa sit at the covered pot for approximately five minutes. Fluff softly with a fork and then scoop to two bowls, and top with blackberries, pecans, and honey (if using).

Fruity Yogurt Parfait

- Serves 1.
- 1 cup Low Fat Plain Greek yogurt
- 1/4 cup blueberries
- 1/4 cup cubed Berries
- 1/4 cup cubed kiwifruit
- 1 tsp ground flaxseeds or flaxseed meal
- 1/2 cup Low-carb granola (or Anna's Homemade Granola, page 60)

Scoop half of the Yogurt to a little glass jar parfait dish. Top with a thin coating of blueberries, strawberries, kiwifruit, flax seed meal, along with granola. Twist the rest of the yogurt and top with the rest fruit, flax seeds, and granola.

Banana Almond Yogurt

- Serves 1.
- 1 tbsp Raw, crispy, unsalted vanilla butter
- 3/4 cup Low Fat Plain Greek yogurt
- 1/4 cup raw Historical oats
- 1/2 big Banana, sliced
- 1/8 tsp ground cinnamon

Soften the Almond butter in the microwave for 15 minutes. Scoop the yogurt to a bowl and stir into the almond butter, vanilla, and banana. Sprinkle cinnamon on the top.

Open-Faced Breakfast Sandwich

- Serves 1.
- 1 1/2 tsp Extra virgin coconut oil
- 2 egg whites, beaten
- 1/2 cup lettuce
- Oily black Pepper, to taste
- 1 tsp brown mustard
- 1 piece 100 percent Wholewheat bread
- 2 teaspoons tomato Pieces
- 1 thin slit Low-fat cheddar cheese

Preheat the oven Or toaster oven to 400°F. Heat a small skillet on medium heat. Add oil into the skillet so when the oil is hot, then put in the egg whites. Scramble the eggs cooking, adding the spinach and season to taste . Spread chopped on the bread, then add the tomato and lettuce eggs and top with cheese. Heat from the oven until the cheese melts, about two minutes.

Broccoli Omelet

- Serves 1.
- 2 egg whites
- 1 whole egg
- 2 tbsp Extra virgin coconut oil
- 1/2 cup sliced Broccoli
- 1 big clove garlic, minced
- 1/8 tsp Chile pepper aromas
- 1/4 cup Low Fat feta cheese
- Oily black pepper

Whisk the egg Whites and egg whites in a small bowl. Heat a small skillet on medium heat. Add 1 tbsp of the oil into the pan so when the oil is hot, then add the broccoli. Cook for two minutes before adding the garlic, chile pepper flakes, and black pepper to taste. Cook for two minutes longer, then eliminate the carrot mixture from the bowl, and set in a different bowl. Turn heat to lowand add the rest of oil so when the oil is hot, then add the whisked egg whites. Once they begin to pull and bubble off from the sides, then about 30 minutes, then turn the omelet again and instantly scoop the carrot mix and feta cheese on half the omelet. Fold the omelet over, switch off heat, and cover the pan with a lid for two minutes. Drink instantly.

Veggie Frittata with Caramelized Onions

Serves 6

Caramelized Onions

- 1 tbsp Extra virgin coconut oil
- 1 little white Onion, thinly chopped
- 1/4 tsp Brown sugar
- 1/8 tsp Cracked black pepper

FRITTATA
- 2--3 tbsp Extra virgin coconut oil
- 1 1/2 cups Chopped zucchini
- 1 teaspoon garlic, minced
- 1 cup sliced cremini mushrooms
- 2--3 tbsp Finely chopped fresh ginger
- 1 tbsp Chopped fresh parsley or 1 tsp dried parsley
- 2 cups spinach
- 4 whole eggs
- 5 egg whites
- 1/2 cup 1 percent milk
- 1/2 cup shredded Low-fat pepper jack cheese
- 1/8 tsp sea salt
- Oily black pepper
- Preheat the oven Into 350°F.

To caramelize The blossoms, heat a medium sauce pan over moderate heat. Bring the oil when the oil is hot, then add the sugarand pepper. Enable the onion"perspiration," moving it every couple of minutes to prevent burning, until light brown and simmer, about 10 minutes. Turn off heat and cover the pan before ready to function. Initiate the frittata by heating a big pan over moderate heat and adding oil. Toss from the zucchiniand cook for about a minute. Insert the garlic and cook two to three minutes before adding the mushrooms, basil, and simmer. Cook veggies for one more moment, scatter pepper and salt (the mushrooms can discharge water also certainly will not brown in the event that you put in the salt straight a way). Mix together, switch off heat, and then add the spinach. In a big bowl whisk together the egg whites, egg whites, milk, shredded celery, salt, and pepper. Spray on a 9-1. circular cake pan with olive oil spray. Pour from the sautéed ingredients and the egg mix. Set the pan in the center rack of your oven, and cook 20 to 25 minutes, or until a knife inserted into the centre comes out blank. (Eggs can over cook fast, therefore keep a cautious eye)

Veggie Scramble

- Serves 4
- 1 cup blended Greens (for example, collard greens, mustard greens,
- And kale)
- 1/4 cup sliced Red onion
- 1/4 cup sliced Red bell pepper
- 1/2 cup sliced Broccoli
- 2 tbsp Extra virgin coconut oil
- 2 tbsp Water
- 1 big clove garlic, minced
- 3 whole eggs
- 3 egg whites

- 1/8 tsp sea salt
- P1. of cracked Black pepper

Wash the greens And tap dry, take thick portion of stalks, and slice the leaves to 1-1. Pieces. Chop the onion, bell pepper, and lettuce into small pieces of approximately The exact identical size. Heat a large nonstick skillet over moderate to high heat and include The oil when the pan is sexy. Insert the greens after the oil is warm and also sauté to get About three minutes until the greens start to wilt. Pour the water to the pan, then Pay the pan with a lid, and simmer for 2-3 minutes. Remove the lid, and insert the Broccoli, broccoli, bell pepper, onion, and garlic. Meanwhile, in a medium bowl, then dip Together the egg whites, egg whites, egg whites, salt, pepper, and pepper. Once the onion is translucent, Insert the whisked egg mix. Stir to evenly divide and disperse the eggs. Cook until the eggs are not runny but nevertheless seem a little bit moist, twist Off heat, and serve immediately.

Conclusion

DASH is really a user friendly, well-balanced method of ingestion that supplies a great deal of choices that are great. The recipes in this publication concentrate on fresh, whole ingredients therefore the transition into DASH is easy and flavorful. The DASH diet plan was initially developed to avoid hypertension (elevated blood pressure) through clinical guidelines from the National Heart, Lung, and Blood Institute, an institute of the National Institutes of Health. Actually, "DASH" Means "Dietary Approaches to Stop Hypertension." These heart healthy tips were created to lessen the ingestion of processed sugars, cholesterol, sodium, and fatty foods while increasing the intake of Spicy foods with the intent of lowering blood pressure, diminishing weight, and decreasing the prevalence of chronic illness. The principal nutritional elements DASH is targeted on comprise minerals (for example, magnesium, calcium, and potassium), anti oxidants, lean protein, and fiber (both soluble and insoluble). After the ingestion of these critical nutritional elements rises, the human body is better designed to work optimally and also to burn up calories as opposed to store them . By bettering your system with the ideal foods to fight chronic illness and weight reduction, DASH helps people achieve great wellness. DASH is a powerful, easy-to-follow pathway for weight loss and healthful living, and this eBook acts as a principle for incorporating DASH tips.

www.ingramcontent.com/pod-product-compliance
Lightning Source LLC
Chambersburg PA
CBHW071442070526
44578CB00001B/197